STRONGER THAN
STIGMA

A CALL TO ACTION: STORIES OF GRIEF, LOSS, AND INSPIRATION!

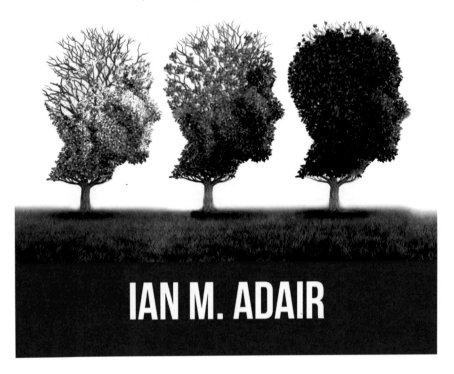

IAN M. ADAIR

1.888.5069-NOW
www.nowscpress.com
@nowscpress

Ordering Information:

   Quantity sales. Special discounts are available on quantity purchases by corporations, associations, and others. For details, contact the publisher at the address above.

   Orders by U.S. trade bookstores and wholesalers. Please contact: NOW SC Press: Tel: (888) 5069-NOW or visit www.nowscpress.com.

Printed in the United States of America

First Printing, 2020

ISBN: 978-1-7341809-8-5

Disclaimer: The information provided in this book is not intended to be a substitute for professional medical advice, diagnosis or treatment that can be provided by your own Medical Provider (including doctor/physician, nurse, physician's assistant, or any other health professional), Mental Health Provider (including psychiatrist, psychologist, therapist, counselor, or social worker), or member of the clergy. Therefore, do not disregard or delay seeking professional medical, mental health or religious advice because of information you have read in this book. Do not stop taking any medications without speaking to your own Medical Provider or Mental Health Provider. If you have or suspect that you or someone you love has a medical or mental health problem, contact your own Medical Provider or Mental Health Provider promptly.

100% of the proceeds from the sale of this book will benefit the Gracepoint Foundation.

Dedication

This book is dedicated to all the courageous and inspiring people who are in recovery, managing a mental health condition, or who have experienced profound grief and loss. To all of the individuals and families who were able to navigate the tragedy of loss and turned that sadness into purpose and action: *Your VOICE* changes the discussion around mental health and addiction. *Your EFFORTS* help eliminate the stigma associated with mental illness and recovery and *Your ACTIONS* save lives every day. This book is for you!

I would like to take the opportunity to express my gratitude to all the mental health professionals, care givers, and advocates out there who support and champion the millions of people suffering from mental illness and addiction every day. Your efforts, work ethic, and kindness are seldom recognized but—to so many of us who suffer or are in recovery—you are our heroes!

To anyone struggling right now with addiction, mental illness, or suicidal thoughts—you are brave, you are strong, and you will get through this. You are not alone.

Contents

Introduction

What makes mental illness so scary for so many people is that we can't see it. It's an invisible disease that anyone can succumb to and suffer from. None of us can predict how we might respond if we lost a loved one, witnessed an atrocity, or suffered a traumatic experience. Then there is the fact that some of us are biologically predisposed to mental illness and addiction if it is in our family medical history.

What is a mental health disorder? It is a diagnosable condition affecting an individual's mood, thinking, or behavior. There is a wide range of mental health disorders. Some of the most common include anxiety, depression, bipolar disorder, schizophrenia, obsessive-compulsive disorder (OCD), substance abuse, and post-traumatic stress disorder (PTSD).

Mental health awareness and addiction have become trending topics in today's news cycle and on social media due to the number of traumatic and negative events. Unfortunately, it has also taken the high-profile suicide deaths of people like Robin Williams, Kate Spade, and Anthony Bourdain, to name a few, to have a greater dialogue around mental illness. What has also pushed the conversation further are the increasing number of professional athletes and celebrities coming out about their battles with depression, anxiety, and addiction. Although this has helped, there is more public sympathy and acceptance given to celebrities and athletes because we almost expect them to make mistakes, develop an addiction, or collapse under the intense public pressure they experience.

Over the last few years, the conversation around mental illness and addiction has become more open and public, but where the discussion is still falling short concerns the stigma faced by many who are not in the public eye or well known. I believe that regular people, those of us not in the public eye, still have a long way to go before we are comfortable with openly disclosing a mental illness or addiction without fear of any consequences or judgment.

Everyday people—working professionals, retired seniors, and students alike—if they disclose a mental illness or addiction fear losing the three things that matter the most to them in their life: their family, their friends, and their job! Disclosing a mental illness or addiction shouldn't mean giving anything up or losing those who should be supporting you but, for many, that fear is real.

The fear so many people face about sharing their battles has been perpetuated by a number of falsehoods, misrepresentations, and myths about mental illness, which prevent many who do suffer from seeking help. There are several myths about mental health (many will come up again in the personal stories shared later in this book), but I believe the following are six of the biggest myths about mental illness that need to be addressed now:

- Myth #1: Mental illness is caused by weakness.
- Myth #2: Mental illness is an excuse for laziness.
- Myth #3: You can feel better whenever you want.
- Myth #4: People can choose to be mentally ill.
- Myth #5: Mental illness is all in someone's head.
- Myth #6: Mental illness really is not that different from feeling sad.

These myths have added to the powerful stigma now attributed to mental illness and addiction while at the same time criticize and diminish those suffering. Mental illness is a treatable disease. For some, diagnosed treatment has a high rate of success; depression being the most treatable. Yet, stigma alone keeps many from getting help and sometimes suffering in silence for years—that is why these myths are so dangerous.

Mental illness and treatment options can be a complex subject matter to understand. For the sake of this book, I want to touch on just a couple of things but also acknowledge that many people reading may be seeing this information for the first time. So we'll start with some explanations: mental illness can only be diagnosed following a thorough assessment and screening by a qualified mental health professional, such as a psychiatrist, psychologist, counselor, or clinical social worker. A wide range of therapies may be used to treat mental health disorders and, depending on the specific issue, some of these therapies include:

- **Psychotherapy.** This includes individual counseling with a private therapist or group therapy. Psychotherapy can help you uncover and work through specific challenges or events in your life that may have contributed to mental illness as well as teach you improved coping skills.

- **Behavioral therapies.** You may participate in cognitive behavioral therapy to address negative, unhealthy thought patterns and make positive changes to behavior, or dialectical behavior therapy, which is often used to help people who have borderline personality disorder or suicidal behavior.

- **Medication.** Different medications are prescribed for various mental illnesses. For example, certain antidepressants are helpful in the treatment of both depression and anxiety. Medications are usually used in conjunction with psychotherapy for the best results.

One of the best ways to break down stigma is by listening to and reading stories of lived experiences. Stories have the ability to impact us on a profound level, especially when we feel a strong connection to the storyteller. Words like *mental illness, addiction, suicide, abuse, profound grief* and *loss* can immediately change a life—forever. For those who suffer in silence, this can be a life or death issue. These myths must be debunked whenever possible so the correct education and awareness can support a person's path to wellness and recovery.

The Climate Today Around Mental Health

This book project began right when the COVID-19 pandemic dominated the news in early February of 2020. Over the months that followed, people started to deal with the realities of social distancing, remote work, quarantine, and isolation. Fear of exposure to the virus and a steadily climbing death toll placed mental health and self-care front and center on all media outlets. For many, being isolated from loved ones and unable to connect with friends and coworkers was not a healthy experience. If anything, what experiencing isolation and social distancing did accomplish was to help people better understand the realities that many living with mental illness face everyday.

The pandemic and the ensuing financial crisis continues to elevate the discussion about mental health. Both the corporate and nonprofit sector have been slow to adopt flexible work schedules and remote working options for their employees, despite the demand. Through this crisis, we have learned that people can be very productive and efficient when working remotely, in most cases working more than normal, but it does take a toll on their mental health.

Research is showing people are working longer, without breaks, and seem more stressed about their jobs because of the stigma of remote work—in other words, they feel they have to be available and working all the time. The lack of connectedness and the fact that many have become emotionally distant, as well as socially distant, caused an increase in number of people who felt depressed and anxious—increasing the need for more mental health services.

How Stronger Than Stigma Started

The Gracepoint Foundation is the philanthropic arm of Gracepoint, one of the largest behavioral health organizations in the state of Florida. The Foundation struggled to gain traction for many years, even though many of the pieces essential to a nonprofit's success were in place. We needed a new strategy to engage the greater Tampa community, especially with those who had a connection to our mission. After meeting with our board of directors, donors, staff, and others from the private sector, our new strategy became obvious—we would embrace and run towards addressing adult mental illness, not away from it.

What we missed was right in front of us: mental illness and addiction impact thousands of people in our community every year and in a variety of ways. We realized that stigma was even affecting the way we fundraised, put on events, and shared our story. Our new focus would be to drive awareness around adult mental health, recognize those in the industry for their work, and create a safe space for people to talk openly about mental illness and addiction.

The idea for this book originated from the success of an event put on by the Gracepoint Foundation, called Stronger Than Stigma. We discussed the idea with many people who did not think an event solely focused on adult mental illness was the best idea. There were real concerns about our ability to raise money and whether or not we could even get people to attend. We learned so much those first two years, but mostly that the Tampa Bay region was ready to talk about and address mental health in a meaningful way. The personal stories shared resonated with our audiences and helped them better understand the power stigma has over people suffering. The event also allowed attendees to find an outlet to share their stories and many sought out the Foundation to get more involved.

According to the Centers for Disease Control and Prevention (CDC), suicide is the number two cause of death for people between the ages of ten and thirty-four and is the fourth leading cause of death among individuals between the ages of thirty-five and fifty-four, yet mental illness is rarely mentioned in the news. One of the biggest factors I believe keeping the general public from understanding the importance of mental health and addiction is the messaging and outreach used by the mental health sector. All the national awareness organizations promote the same statistic—that one in five adults in America will experience a diagnosable mental illness in a given year. What they forget to promote is that *five out of five* people have mental health and, by forgetting this, they discount the connection all of us have with anyone who has suffered from mental illness or addiction or is suffering today.

Whenever I speak about mental health to any group, I always ask the audience to raise their hand if they personally, a member of their family, or someone in their inner circle of closest friends has ever been impacted by mental illness, suicide, or addiction. Each time I ask this question, almost every single person in the room raises their hand. If we all have mental health or know someone who has struggled, then why are we not promoting the urgency of the issue in a way that shares this connection to better get people's attention?

Two incredibly important incidents happened the week of our first Stronger Than Stigma event, amplifying the importance of mental health and our work in the community. Just two days before the event, it was reported that Kate Spade had died by suicide and, the day after the event, the news broke of Anthony Bourdain's death by suicide. The news regarding both of these important public figures dominated cable and local news around the world. Mental health, addiction, and suicide were all trending topics on social media for weeks to follow. Here were two very successful people, whose names were recognizable to almost everyone—both suffered privately and had just ended their lives. Not since the death of Robin Williams had the media focused so much on the topic of mental health and suicide.

Our event, by all measure, was a success. It didn't raise the most money or draw the largest crowd but we felt we succeeded in getting the most compelling message out for this first time as an organization. We found our audience connected better with the stories of lived experience and witnessed how those stories helped break down stigma. We learned that stigma is a very broad issue that cannot be addressed in only one way. We realized we could confront stigma from many perspectives and raise more awareness by allowing people with different experiences to share their mental illness and addiction stories.

About the Stories Included in This Book

One of the best ways to educate about stigma is to acknowledge the context people apply when discussing mental illness and addiction. Mental illness and addiction can impact any person regardless of gender, sexuality, race, or socioeconomic status, in other words— everyone. The stories shared in this book are from successful people, in their chosen field, who have lived through extraordinary circumstances. I want readers to get to know them as authentic people who have lives outside of their chosen professional world. People who have struggled with problems and yet, figured out how to help and serve others.

For this book I wanted to address stigma through this collection of stories, because stories have the power to connect us to one another. Stories are the common ground that allow people to communicate and overcome our differences so we can better understand ourselves and each other. Through story we can see the world through someone else's eyes and emotionally connect with their situation. Because of this, stories are powerful tools—and it takes powerful tools to fight and end stigma.

Our Stronger Than Stigma event taught us that our audience connected with our speakers through their shared story. These personal stories have helped hundreds to understand the power stigma has over those suffering—how it prevents people from seeking help and even prevents them from sharing their struggles with family or friends. My hope for this book is to help even more people through these twelve powerful stories of hope, recovery, and inspiration.

I have two main goals for this book. The first, to share stories from a variety of perspectives that include: caregivers, suicide survivors, those who have experienced profound grief and loss, victims of abuse, and people who manage their mental illness and recovery every day. Second, I want to inspire people to take action and get involved. The storytellers in this book all fall into one or more of the following categories: They are actively involved in supporting mental health and addiction awareness, passionate about sharing their story to inspire others, and support efforts to improve the quality of life of those suffering.

Through a series of interviews and discussions each storyteller shares how they process their grief and loss, as well as how they diligently and carefully manage their addiction, mental illness, and self-care. The following stories are written in the first person and set up in such a way so you, the reader, make a connection with the storyteller. Each chapter is broken into three subsections: My Story, Path to Wellness and Recovery, and a Call to Action. I end each chapter by sharing how each person is actively involved in helping others, sharing their story, ending stigma, and changing the conversation around mental health to be more open and supportive.

The first step towards action is having a conversation. I hope these stories start the critical and essential conversations needed in this country around mental health and addiction so that anyone suffering feels safe to disclose a challenge and get the help they need. As storytellers, we hold the power to shape narratives and influence what people think is possible. We have to lean into that power when it concerns mental health and addiction, use it to not only address stigma, but to eliminate it altogether.

In the stories you are about to read, this amazing group of people share their sadness, hardships, and joys—but most of all, their purpose.

Ben Heldfond

Entrepreneur / Investor / Owner, Heldfond Holdings

Need hadn't motivated me to go to the meetings. Need hadn't encouraged me to be honest. Need hadn't made me resist the urge to use. Want, however, did. I wanted to stop living my life like that and I wanted to stop the incomprehensible demoralization I felt every single day.

My Story

I was talking to my ex-girlfriend on the phone one night as I was shooting heroin. It was 1993, long before cell phones, so I was on a landline. The next thing I know, she's standing over me. The door to my house had been knocked down and paramedics were working on me. I had overdosed while I was on the phone. Landlines, unlike cell phones just don't drop calls, she knew something wasn't right and was able to save my life. Every time a call has dropped in the years since, I have thought about that day and how a simple landline is responsible for my being here today.

I had been held back in kindergarten and my "flunking" kindergarten became a joke. It was the first time in my life I remember feeling less than or that I was different than the other kids. Then in third grade, I remember hearing, "there's something wrong with Ben" which was the first time I heard those words. I was soon diagnosed with dyslexia and ADHD. I remember sitting in class and not understanding things as quickly as the other kids. My mind didn't quite get it, then I'd beat myself up and think I was just dumb. Daydreaming became my first drug of choice because I could check out and not worry about anything.

I was born and raised in San Francisco by parents who were very young when they got married. They divorced when I was thirteen in a typical high conflict fashion, their battle became a tough place for a kid with super-low self-esteem to live. I had already been experimenting with drugs and alcohol, and the tension at home just gave me an excuse to accelerate my using.

A lot of teenagers are like water, they are able to find the weakest point, I was no different. I played one parent off the other and used that to my advantage. If my mom made my curfew earlier, my dad would make it later. If Mom gave me ten dollars then Dad would give me twenty. For as long as I can remember, I tried to take a shortcut to get what I wanted. Whenever I got into trouble, my parents rushed to get me out of it so I never really faced any consequences for my actions. I went through life with this feeling of invincibility and entitlement.

At my high school graduation, I was high on psychedelic drugs. My diploma was blank when they handed it to me and I couldn't tell if that was a real piece of paper or if the LSD was making me see things. I didn't deal with anything—school, pressure or the divorce—in healthy or productive ways. I used drugs and alcohol to self-medicate and I got very good at figuring out what combination numbed my pain the best.

At Berkeley, I was recruited as a goaltender for the soccer team. At my third practice, the coach pulled me aside and said the current goalie was a sophomore so I wouldn't be seeing much playing time until after he graduated. I had an inferiority complex and was not happy about this revelation. I was also an egomaniac, so I was outraged. I told the coach he didn't know who he had recruited and that he was making a terrible mistake. Just to show him, I quit the team.

That moment was a microcosm of my life. I didn't want to put in the work. I wanted the easiest path AROUND the problem or issue instead of putting in the time and going through the problem. I felt entitled to be the starting goalie and quit when I didn't get my way.

I left the field, walked down the main street of Berkeley's Greek row, I walked past a house that I recognized the Greek letters because it was the same Fraternity my brother belonged to at UCLA. Right when I walked in the front door a guy I knew from high school gave me a big bear hug. I put my soccer bag down in the hall and, without taking a moment to think, was snorting a line of cocaine and knocking back a shot of tequila two seconds later. School hadn't even started yet, but I had found my party friends.

> About 25% of people who try heroin will become addicted.
>
> Source: Addiction Center

It did not take long until one of my friends came over with heroin. I knew what it was. I knew what it could do and still, just as before, there was no window between my thought and my action. I smoked it the first time and didn't feel anything. So then I tried injecting it. The second the heroin hit my brain, I felt like I had kissed Jesus. I found everything I had been searching for and, for the first time, my mind wasn't talking back at all. I was nineteen, at the end of my sophomore year in college, and I was a heroin addict.

At Berkeley, since I was a diagnosed dyslexic student, it meant I got special treatment. I received a stipend to hire someone to take notes for me and I was allowed to take untimed, open book tests. This all helped me hold up the façade that I was doing okay in my classes. I even had a decent GPA for quite a while, but the reality of my situation was about to set in.

Up until that time I tried heroin, I had been able to juggle every ball in my life—frat life, school, work, girlfriend, and family. But when I became a daily heroin user, it wasn't long before I was unable to juggle all of the balls in the air. One by one, they began to hit the floor, until there was only one ball left, the addiction ball. The heroin brought me to my knees. Every time I shot up, I was chasing the first kiss from Jesus feeling. No matter how many times I tried, I never found it again.

My family found out that I'd been lying about everything and my mother gave me two choices. "Behind door number one," she said, "is support and love if you go to rehab. Behind door number two, there is no support and no more paying your rent." I chose a twenty-eight-day rehab program. The first thing Mike, my counselor at the center, said to me was "recovery is a pretty simple program, all you have to do is change your whole life." I wasn't ready to change my whole life and, in that moment, my relapse started.

I was nicknamed the "everything's cool guy" in my recovery program. I was great at bullshitting other people, using some of the nuggets I'd picked up in the twelve-step program to make it sound like I had everything together. I got out and went back to Berkeley, even though I had been kicked out of school. I had lied to my parents and told them I was just going to take a semester off to concentrate on my recovery. Deep down, I knew it was just a matter of time before I relapsed.

Path to Wellness and Recovery

I was at dinner one night and, as soon as I thought about getting high, I immediately left and scored. Once again, there was no barrier between thought and action; no window of time when I paused and to play the movie all the way to the end. I sat there with my needles and drugs, once again alone with my addiction—and it suddenly all became clear. I could see where my life was going and, in that moment, I stopped needing sobriety and switched to *wanting* sobriety.

Need hadn't motivated me to go to the meetings. Need hadn't encouraged me to be honest. Need hadn't made me resist the urge to use. Want, however, did. I wanted to stop living my life like that and I wanted to stop the incomprehensible demoralization I felt every single day.

The first step to dealing with addiction is admitting that you are powerless and that your life is unmanageable. I saw myself and what my future would be if I didn't get help through the eyes of other people in the meetings. Any thoughts I ever entertained that this was "just a phase" disappeared and the foundation for the window between thought and action began to grow.

For six months, I'd been going to the rehab center and paying $125 an hour to lie to my counselor. That day, I started our meeting with honesty. Not because I had been caught or that I'd overdosed, but because I wanted to be honest. Mike looked at my mom and said, "Finally." He had known I was lying all that time and he'd also known that nothing would work, no matter what he said, until I found my own way and had my own motivation to get clean.

I went to a medical detox and I freaked out the first day. I told them I didn't want to go to a transition house after detox; that I'd rather die than go. The threat to kill myself meant they had to 5150 me (California code for involuntary psychiatric commitment), complete with a straightjacket and a shot of Thorazine. I was locked up in the psych ward. The other patients were going about their normal business, watching TV and playing cards—except there was no TV and there weren't any cards on the table. It was a moment straight out of the movie *One Flew Over the Cuckoo's Nest*.

I realized this was where I was going to permanently end up if I didn't get honest with myself. It scared me. I called my mom and begged her to get me out of there. To her credit, she made me stay there for the whole seventy-two hours. It was the first time she had torn off that blanket of codependency and I knew I wasn't going to be able to fool her again. By the end of those three days, I was willing and desperate to come clean. I went through detox and then on to a halfway house. That place was such a great thing to build my sobriety on because it was all about being accountable, something I had never had to be.

The 'Customs and Courtesies' book at the halfway house had rules, on top of rules, on top of rules. If I was late more than three times, I would be kicked out. If I missed a meeting, I would be kicked out. If I lost my job, I would be kicked out. At the time, I was a twenty-one-year-old with an attitude and thought there was no way I could do this, but I did. I stayed sober for six months and never received a single late violation. Those rules were perfect for someone like me, who had been self-centered and had never suffered any consequences.

The three-strike program had just started in California and I saw at least a half a dozen guys get one last chance, mess it up, and then end up in jail for twenty-five years. I was headed down that path and didn't want that life. I began to attend twelve-step meetings with a different attitude—a new blessing of desperation and willingness. I'd look around the room and know that, no matter what looked different between us—our race or age—everything else was the same and I could learn from these people. The three parts of the twelve-step triangle are *service, program, fellowship*, and I realized that, for me, fellowship was the key. I would go to IHOP with the other guys after the meeting and laugh like I'd never laughed before. I enjoyed those moments the most because I was accepted exactly as I was.

The hardest time in my sobriety came when I got divorced. We had a young son and I wish I had an excuse like drinking or using to blame for what happened. We had just moved to Tampa from San Francisco. I had twelve years of sobriety then and felt like I was an old-timer. I went to a few meetings, but missed the fellowship of my old group and didn't like feeling like a newcomer. I stopped going to meetings and,

> About 6% of American adults (about 15 million people) have an alcohol use disorder, but only about 7% of Americans who are addicted to alcohol ever receive treatment.
>
> Source: Addiction Center

instead of being sober and working the program, I was just abstinent from drugs and alcohol.

That misery I was feeling manifested in my relationship and turned me into a dry drunk—I still behaved in dysfunctional ways. I was angry and saw it all as her fault. Everything I had learned about accountability went right out the window.

I hired a big-time lawyer to go after her and I began to read the lawyer's game plan on a plane ride back from Los Angeles. Two pages into this twenty-five-page document, I had a moment of clarity. If I continued down this path, the only person who would get hurt was our son. My parents' divorce and all the tension I'd endured as a kid came to mind and made me see that our anger would be like poison to our son and he'd pay the emotional price. My life had come full circle.

When I landed, I got back to my meetings and took that turning point on the plane as a vow to make this divorce different. Ours could have been like every other horrifying divorce. But, for the grace of God, I was able to tap into the main thing I had learned at the halfway house 13 years prior, accountability and honesty. This along with my past experience of divorce, I was able to not repeat those mistakes.

By going back to the roots of my twelve steps, I could see a different way forward with my ex-wife. I went to ninety meetings in ninety days and worked my steps around what happened during our relationship. I asked her to coffee one day, told her I loved her, apologized to her, and made amends.

Call to Action

Thirteen years later, meeting my ex-wife for coffee set in motion a completely amazing outcome for us which culminated with the writing of *Our Happy Divorce*. Every decision we have made has been through the lens of what's best for our son. Now, we are both remarried to other people and live five houses apart.

I've been sober now for twenty-five years. I can't say I've done it perfectly, but I haven't taken a drink or used. Those first five years of my sobriety built a solid foundation inside me, so when a storm does come along I have a better chance of surviving it. All of us are fighting like hell, every day, not to backslide. That's recovery in a nutshell. We're all just ordinary people who achieved something extraordinary.

I want people to know, those feelings of not being enough are a hole that you are always trying to plug. For years, I tried to fill that hole with addiction before I realized that the only way to fix a spiritual problem is with a spiritual solution. There's nothing else; I've tried it all.

Today, I put some of my time and energy into supporting organizations that help addicts, such as Young People in Recovery, Road Recovery and Phoenix House Florida. These organizations help and impact so many and I encourage everyone I know to get involved if they can.

I'm the co-host of a radio show here in the Tampa Bay area on 102.5 The Bone, called Miggs & Swig—Life Out Loud. I use that platform to share my story, discuss mental health and addiction topics, and to keep the discussion ongoing whenever I can. I want people to understand that there should be the same compassion for people with mental health and addiction challenges as there is for people with cancer. There's power in openness and in telling our stories as a motivator for change.

The thought of using or drinking again never goes away. Even today, twenty-five years later, I know I'm an addict. I still have the same kinds of issues—personal and work related—that could make me turn to drugs or alcohol again. The difference is now I take the right actions in that window of space, whether it's calling someone or going to a meeting, that stop me from returning to that way of life.

Rita Lowman

Bank President / *Tampa Bay Business Journal*'s 2018 Business Woman of the Year

Recovery is a beautiful thing but it also requires daily management and initiative. Both you and your loved ones need positive reinforcement, every day. You have to keep talking and keep the dialogue going. Together, you can get through it.

My Story

The call from the hospital came, my stomach dropped, and every worst fear I'd ever had as a parent rushed in so fast it took me a second to remember to breathe. To move. To act. The doctor started to tell us that we were lucky because our son had overdosed but that he had been saved in time. My eyes opened, all those whispers of doubt in my gut became loud shouts and I recognized this was a serious issue we had denied for too long. I realized two things at the same time: My child was alive, thank God, and he needed serious help.

I remember that moment vividly. The drive to the hospital seemed to take ten years and at the same time, ten seconds. I rushed through the halls and when I reached my son in the emergency room I shuddered to a stop. Our youngest son, the smart, funny, clever child who had once made friends with one of the bulls on our farm, was lying on a table hooked up to machines that beeped a steady reminder of a reality I had been blind to until that very moment.

No one would look at me and my husband—upper middle class, successful executives with a happy family—and think we were going through this kind of thing. You can raise several children in the same house, with a happy family or one that lives in chaos, and have a different outcome for each child. Our family was in the middle of what others would call a good, full, and ordinary life. Two grown sons, a long and happy marriage, and successful careers. We thought we were doing great—until that moment when the phone rang and the nurse's tone told us things were bad and that our son was in real trouble.

Clint was our second born son. Growing up, he always struggled with anxiety. Up to that point, he had been acting a little off but I had chalked it up to late-teens behavior. Those are the years when kids rebel, hide away in their rooms a little more, and want to be anywhere but in a room with mom and dad.

We had enabled him in some ways, but there's a thin line you tread as a parent between care and codependency. When Clint was in high school and he'd ask me for twenty dollars, I'd give him the money without thinking about it. I'd assume he was spending it on food or gas or a girl, not his addiction. In hindsight, I shouldn't have been giving him cash but I loved him and believed him when he told me why he needed the money.

I didn't have any answers, no one really did in those days, and it was such a taboo subject to talk about twenty years ago. I didn't know anyone else who had a child with addiction and mental health issues. Not because they didn't exist but, if other people were going through the same thing, they weren't sharing their pain, their fears, or their advice. I had never witnessed something like this, never had to deal with it, and, even though my husband and I had achieved great things professionally, in that moment I felt more inept than I had ever felt before.

> About 20% of Americans who have depression or an anxiety disorder also have a substance use disorder.
>
> Source: Addiction Center

I had to learn to ask the questions, do the research, and to talk to anyone I could. I leaned on my husband and my faith. I knew that if God had brought my son through this, then He had a reason and a purpose for him. It would be another two decades before that purpose was realized. Those years would be filled with wonderful highs, chased by lows so deep they nearly broke us.

On the dark days, I would remind myself of the old adage that God never gives us more than we can bear; even if, in that moment, we didn't think we could possibly carry that weight for one more second. On brighter days, I reminded my son how loved and precious he was. And in between all of it, I prayed.

My son is brilliant and I've heard him have some of the most amazing conversations with other people. Along with that brilliance came some depression and anxiety, but I thought what he was going through was normal and would eventually sort itself out. I would ask him if he was okay and he'd say he was fine. And I believed him until that day in the hospital, when I realized he had a serious problem with his mental health and addiction.

If you're a parent with a child who is battling mental illness or addiction, you have to open your eyes and recognize what is happening. I didn't open my eyes soon enough. Our child was suffering but, in reality, the entire family was suffering.

Path to Wellness and Recovery

We had to learn the hard way that most people who suffer with addiction don't recover after one visit to a rehab facility and not every mental illness improves after the first course of treatment or counseling. Many people need two or three stays in a facility and have to try several combinations of medications before they can finally start the recovery process. I know the tendency is to push someone who is hurting toward recovery and I know how hard it is to wait for your loved one to be ready for help. If they aren't ready, the chances of relapse are very high.

It was traumatic in different ways and on different levels for each one of us. My husband and I had to deal with feelings of guilt and thousands of what ifs. We spent many nights unable to sleep, pacing the floors, worried and scared. It took a long time until we realized that we didn't cause it, and we can't cure it or control it.

I have wished, a million times, that I could go back and change the past, but that's impossible. What I can do—what any parent can do—is be there and be present right now. I talk to him every day and tell him how much I love him. Even when things were at their worst, my message was the same—*I love you and I'm here.*

You have to talk to the people around you. Unfortunately, sometimes those closest to you will often say what you want to hear, instead of the truth. A good friend will not just be a sounding board, but a dose of reality. Even though people think I'm an extrovert, I tend to internalize a lot of things. I have a very good friend I rely on and I also have my husband. He has been the amazing powerhouse behind helping our son and keeping our family strong. I've kept a journal for decades and writing down what I was going through all those years has helped me.

Over the years my best advice from it all is: Don't block yourself off from the world. Talk to a friend or a therapist. Find a support group. You are definitely not the only parent that has gone through this. It takes a village, as they say, and everyone needs a village to help them. We have each other and I am very grateful for that. When my husband and I realized our son was not healthy, mentally or physically, we began to look at options to help him get well. For us, it was a family initiative. I have such sympathy for people who are struggling to find help alone because they often feel judged and isolated. Mental illness is as much of a real illness as addiction, cancer, or anything else.

> Almost 21 million Americans have at least one addiction, yet only 10% of them receive treatment.
>
> Source: Addiction Center

The hardest thing to accept is that sometimes the person you love isn't ready to get help. You can't give up on them. I've met parents who said it wasn't worth their time to keep talking to their child suffering from addiction because they had stopped listening. I want to tell every parent that it is worth your time! It is worth every single word you say. You don't want to be a member of the other group of parents I have met—the ones whose children have taken that last, fatal step and are no longer here. Those parents would gladly sacrifice everything they have to try one more time to get their child help. Don't stop having those conversations. Don't ever stop.

Call to Action

There is no stereotypical family with a child who struggles with addiction and mental health challenges—it happens in every kind of family. That's exactly why I talk about what our family went through— to tell other parents that you aren't alone and that you need support as much as the person you love does.

This is not an easy road, not for the family and not for the person who needs help. Recovery is a beautiful thing but it also requires daily management and initiative. Both you and your loved one need positive reinforcement every day. You have to keep talking and keep the dialogue going. Together, you can get through it.

I encourage parents to look for those first signs, even if they don't know what those signs might be. If your child is in their room all the time, talking too fast, not making coherent statements, maybe eating too much, too little or too many sweets, those could all be indications that things aren't what they seem. When something is different in your child's life, ask questions. Talk to them. Don't be afraid to confront them about whatever is going on, and whatever you do, don't turn a blind eye. Your loved one may need your help, maybe more than you know.

I'll never stop worrying that the phone is going to ring at 2:00 a.m. After everything we have been through, our family has made it a mission to stay close to each other. Those are the people you can depend upon and will help you get through life. Keep them near and keep the communication going.

Look around you. There are people you meet every day whose lives are touched by someone with mental illness or addiction. We need to keep having these difficult conversations. Most of all, keep fighting with legislators and insurance companies to get the support and resources people need. We also need better resources for those suffering and facilities for treatment.

Every night, before my husband and I fall asleep, we send our son a simple text: *I love you. Have a good night.* My heart catches in the minutes I wait until he sends back, *I love you too.* And when I close my eyes, I hope he knows that I'm still saying, *I love you and I'm here for you. Always.*

I want people to know we have to keep talking to, keep supporting, and keep loving that person in our life who is struggling. You can never take too many steps to help someone you love. I'm working hard to encourage emerging leaders and the next generation to be positive role models who are open and honest about their own challenges. Together we are stronger.

Less than a month after my interview for this book, on February 26, 2020, my son Clinton Hooper Lowman passed away.

After almost two years of sobriety and staying clean, his life was finally on the right track. The medical report came back that Clint passed away due to a weak heart. The condition was consistent with heart conditions in my family medical history—both my maternal great grandfather and grandfather also had it.

I am still receiving text messages and emails from the many lives Clint touched over the years. His desire to help others overcome their problems was evident in his willingness to work in the mental health and addiction field. He was a rock for those suffering and needing inspiration to get help. These testimonials have been incredible for us to hear and have helped us through our grieving process.

I simply cannot thank everyone in our lives who has passed on their thoughtful messages and prayers to our family for the loss of my beautiful son.

Jason Caras

CEO and Co-Chairman of the Board, IT Authorities

Depression is a lot more than feeling down, it is a powerful emotional state that can drive us to think and do the unthinkable. Suffering in silence can lead to shame, severe depression, or even suicide. If we are open and honest about negative feelings and emotions, we take away the power they can have over us, making it easier to reach out for help.

My Story

I remember when I started taking real risks with my life. I would come home from school, grab my father's 357 Magnum, sit on the edge of his bed, and hold it up to my head. I would sit there for a half an hour, just thinking, contemplating suicide. Every time, I would put the gun back. There was something inside me that was hanging on, that still had some hope.

My bipolar disorder, although undiagnosed at the time, mostly came in the form of mania. I was always willing to risk more, to leave it all out there, and to give whatever I was doing everything I had. I was incredibly intense when I was young. That mania found an outlet in hockey. I became a brutally rough hockey player because it was a way to get my anger out. I also channeled some of that mania into being an entrepreneur. I was selling things door to door and had already started a couple of businesses before I graduated high school.

I started using drugs and alcohol to self-medicate. I was always trying to chase the next level I could reach. I drove like an absolute maniac, which often resulted in epic police chases. I was arrested nine times before I turned seventeen. I lived in this hyper-perpetual manic state until I crashed, which didn't happen as often as the mania when I was growing up. I attempted suicide for the first time when I was twelve. My parents were going through a divorce. I was angry. I went out on my motorcycle and tried to get hit by a car on purpose. Somehow, I survived, but everything I did at that time was with whirlwind intensity.

As an adult, that intensity continued. I started businesses over

> Bipolar disorder affects approximately 5.7 million adult Americans, or about 2.6% of the U.S. population age 18 and older every year. (National Institute of Mental Health)
>
> Source: Depression and Bipolar Support Alliance

and over again. I still had that risk-taking mentality and went on to jeopardize everything I owned three different times. In my mind, I was willing to do and risk what others would not to be successful. This behavior translated to relationships, as well. I loved the idea of falling in love and glamorizing somebody, but then I was done with that person in three or four weeks. It got to the point where even my close friends would say, "I love him but you shouldn't date him."

In my early thirties, I crashed harder than ever. I had been heavily self-medicating, mainly with alcohol, and my latest business venture had just cost me everything I owned. I was disgusted with myself, with my life, and with everything I was going through. I was in a car with my friend and I tried to jump out of it while she was going eighty miles an hour on the highway. She suggested I go to Alcoholics Anonymous and, when I got there, the manic part of me figured I could get through that program in one day. I went eighteen months without drinking, but I was bored silly because things weren't as fun as when I was drinking. Every time I got like that, I convinced myself that I was bored with my life.

I told myself it wasn't depression, but it was and I knew it. I remember having conversations with people and, in my head, I was having my last conversation ever with them because I was going to kill myself that day. Then I wouldn't go through with it. I'd start to come out of the depression and regain my 'fighting for my life' kind of attitude.

When I was thirty-two, I went to see a doctor who immediately had me pegged. She knew right away I was suffering from bipolar disorder. I got so upset that she figured me out so quickly and I thought she was just a pill pusher. I was in denial that anything was wrong with me, even though I had suicidal thoughts on several occasions since I was twelve years old. I walked away from her and went back to self-medicating and living in a primarily manic state. I was self-destructive and had bouts of severe depression. It would be another ten years before I went to another doctor.

Path to Wellness and Recovery

I was on an emotional roller coaster for almost four decades. I knew there had to be more to life than this constant internal battle. I decided to get help, but this time I would keep an open mind.

I found a doctor who specializes in forensic psychology. She confirmed that I had bipolar disorder and spent two hours listening to me talk about how I felt. I remembered she pointed to a cup on the table and said, "Up here, on the top is mania, and down on the bottom is depression—where are you?" I told her I was in the middle. "No, you're manic now," she said. I insisted I was in the middle, right between the two, but I knew she knew better.

My doctor started trying me on different medications. The first two or three she prescribed really didn't work, but she convinced me to be patient and try different drug combinations. I was put on Zyprexa and felt like I was in the middle (between mania and depression) for the first time ever. I wasn't, but I didn't realize that until I slowly sank into a really long depression that lasted for weeks. Then she added ten milligrams of Prozac to my prescription and that was when the illumination happened and everything changed.

For the first time in my life, I felt like there was something controlling the angry outbursts and the manic side of my bipolar disorder. Over the years, she and I have tweaked and changed the dosages as needed. I've learned that this illness requires consistent daily management and that there is no immediate or permanent fix.

One of the biggest issues with bipolar disorder is the desire to get off of the medicine you're taking because you don't feel like yourself. This happens when you are not taking the right combination or correct dosages for you. The meds can make you feel dialed down too much and a shell of yourself. But when the combination is correct, like it finally became for me, it was like a million light bulbs going off and I found a clarity I never previously experienced.

Now that I'm medicated, I can handle any level of bad news and emergency. The medicine does not get a hundred percent of the credit, but it does help me manage my feelings and deal with whatever comes my way. Even though I own and run a large business with a hundred employees, I feel I can handle the obstacles and challenges thrown my way.

I'm grateful, every day, that I've been able to tame the roller coaster in my head and manage my anxiety and depression. I've stopped self-medicating with substances and I love life now, whether it's a good day or a bad day. That's what I want for other people with bipolar disorder to experience—I want them to love their lives, too.

Today, I live a life of gratitude. I use gratitude in moments of reflection, not only at the end of each day but also for helping me manage the impulses that would lead me away from my goals. Consistency has been my key to make this happen. I practice putting distance (ten seconds at least) between when I have an impulse and taking any action. I take some extra time when I have thoughts about drinking or self-medicating to get out of a depressive state, and by doing so the urge usually subsides. Even though my mind says "This will make you feel better," I know that it won't after a few seconds.

I don't live a drink-free life, but I also don't use it as a crutch or as an escape. If something angers me or has the potential to put me over the edge, I take a few minutes to allow it to go through my body and mind and then release it. This coping mechanism takes practice and time, but I find myself calmer at the end of the exercise.

Discipline is another trait I try to strengthen each and every day. My consistent adherence to my disciplines (routines and self-care) allow me to plow through so much bad head noise and any temptations. When I create a discipline, or adhere to one, I feel a sense of accomplishment, which then transcends into increased self-esteem and self-confidence. This self-imposed discipline is powerful; it is my offense and my defense, and very much part of the daily management of my mental illness.

Call to Action

As soon as I saw the change that medication made in my life, I knew that I needed to help others suffering from bipolar disorder get help. I encourage them to keep going, to keep trying different combinations of medicine. I'm real with them and remind them that it's going to suck before it gets better. I reassure them that you eventually get to a good place; it just takes patience. The fact is that your life completely changes when you are properly medicated, giving you an opportunity to write yourself a new story.

Generally speaking, I am on blast about my mental health condition, which just means I am an open book and more than happy to share anything. Although I'm generally a private person, when it comes to mental health, I don't hold back. I'm not afraid to put my battles with my own mental illness on full display. One of the biggest problems today concerning mental health is we avoid talking about it. I know there are good reasons for this, but I believe the only way to fight the stigma associated with mental health is to be open about our stories and struggles.

As many as 1 in 5 patients with bipolar disorder completes suicide.

Source: Depression and Bipolar Support Alliance

I try to share with everyone I know that mental health is no different than physical health and that we need to be more open about it. Suffering in silence can lead to shame, severe depression, or even suicide. Depression is a lot more than feeling down; it is a powerful emotional state that can drive us to think and do the unthinkable. If we are open and honest about negative feelings and emotions, we take away the power they can have over us, making it easier to reach out for help.

Because of my extraordinary openness about my mental health issues, I have been contacted by countless people to talk to their loved ones about my process. I speak to young people, between the ages of twelve and eighteen, who are in the juvenile justice and foster care system or returning to society from the juvenile system. Many of them have suffered from an undiagnosed mental illness their whole lives, which has led to addiction issues and incidents with the law. I share my mental health journey with them to show them that it's okay to have a mental illness and not be embarrassed by it, and to educate them that mental health is a part of life for everyone.

I also coach kids one on one and help them get the medical and psychiatric assistance they may need. I educate them about the process of finding the right medication or combination of medications. I encourage patience because it is key. It can take years to get your mental health dialed in properly.

I used to be embarrassed to admit I have bipolar disorder, now I proudly tell people and share that it can be controlled with medicine, good diet, and healthy habits. I like to think I'm helping change people's lives for the better and that I make a difference in the world. Helping others, I have found, positively impacts my own mental wellbeing and I don't plan on ever stopping.

Today, I truly believe my bipolar disorder is a superpower. I thank God I didn't take my life on those occasions when I was at my lowest. I continue to find ways to spread awareness about mental health anyway I can, whether on a stage, one on one, or through social and digital media. The more people who understand mental health is just as important as physical health, and that there is no shame in having a mental illness, then perhaps suicide can be prevented.

If you—or someone you know—suffer from any type of mental illness, I strongly encourage you to contact a mental health professional near you so you can get the help you need. I did and it saved my life.

Spiros Vassilakos

President, Athenian
Private Client Group

So many young people today are growing up in multicultural and multiethnic households, like I did, where addiction and mental illness are prevalent. If my story can help them, I'm happy to share it.

My Story

As I entered the hospital room, it was clear from the scene of my grieving family that I was too late and my mother had already passed away. I missed the chance to say goodbye. I pulled back the white curtain that was draped in front of the hospital bed where she still lay and knew this would be the last time I would ever see her. Seeing my mom lying there, pale and still, was incredibly hard for me. In that moment, I noticed how peaceful and calm she looked. I had never seen that look before. She had suffered so much, for so long, and even though I was upset, I felt a deep sense of relief that her suffering had finally ended.

It wasn't until right after my mother's death that I realized how bad her drinking had been. Cleaning out her room I found at least a dozen gallon bottles of vodka and gin that were stored under her bed. Gallon bottles! The sheer amount she drank was both incredible and frightening. I believe, to this day, that she gave up and just didn't want to live anymore. I couldn't imagine how she managed to drink so much and function the way she did. But more than that, I couldn't imagine the many years she suffered in silence with this disease.

My mother's daily routine was heartbreaking and that of a classic alcoholic. She got up every morning, went to work, came home to make my brother and I dinner, and then she started drinking. The cycle repeated itself every day for almost three decades. I resigned myself to the fact, long before she died, that if my mother continued drinking she would not live very long. She had other health issues and the drinking only exacerbated them. To me, it was always a matter of time.

To the outside world, she was a productive member of society, not an alcoholic. She was seen as a loving and respected person in the community. A mother who loved her children and someone who welcomed anyone into our home with warmth and a smile. She was the one whom others relied on for advice or who supported them when they were struggling. Despite her drinking, she was the person everyone in the family gravitated toward. So when people came over to visit, which was often, that gave her an excuse to start drinking.

There were times when she really tried to get help. She floated in and out of rehab centers and AA meetings. Sometimes she took me with her to the meetings. I saw how these programs offered hope to my mother, a place where she knew she wasn't alone in her battle with addiction. Her days of sobriety and her relapses were a constant roller coaster. I didn't know what to do, how to help, or how to make her stop before she made the inevitable decision to start drinking again.

My mother shared some of the weight of her pain and heartache with me when I was in college. Her confession of the trauma she had experienced when she was younger helped me understand why she struggled so terribly with alcoholism. Her childhood had been very difficult. Her parents divorced when she was twelve years old and her brothers were in and out of jail—both battled PTSD and drug addiction. But it was when one of her sisters died by suicide in 1968 that impacted and devastated her the most. Her life seemed to be one traumatic event after another. Every time she got sober, something would happen and she would start drinking again.

I believe a series of traumatic events cultivated and supported my mother's alcohol dependence, as well as the time period (1960s) and our Hispanic culture. She was married prior to meeting my father and had two daughters with her first husband but, after years of physical and emotional abuse, she divorced him. People on the Hispanic side of my family never really communicated about

> Approximately 33% of Hispanic or Latinx adults with mental illness receive treatment each year compared to the U.S. average of 43%. This is due to many unique barriers to care. Language Barriers, Less Health Insurance Coverage, Lack of Cultural Competence in providers, Legal Status, Stigma.
>
> Source: National Alliance on Mental Illness

anything, especially their feelings. So alcohol became my mother's preferred method of coping with her trauma and suffering.

The Hispanic side of my family, we're of Puerto Rican descent, was festive and loud, like a constant party. If you were stressed, worried, or depressed, it didn't matter—have a drink and it will all be better. Drinking was such a part of our family's culture that it was hard for anyone to confront it as an actual problem. My uncle, who worked on the police force, was also a functional alcoholic. No one talked about the horrific things he witnessed, the trauma he experienced, or the stress he was under. Maybe that's why no one said anything about my mother's alcoholism, as well.

> According to the National Institute on Alcohol Abuse and Alcoholism, more than 5.3 million women ages 18 and older have an alcohol use disorder.
>
> Source: Talbott Recovery

My father was of Greek heritage, which couldn't have been any more different from my mother's family. The Greek side of my family was very structured and career minded, with everything usually revolving around the work they did. If you owned a restaurant, then the whole family worked there. More importantly, when you were in a social setting with other people, those people were always Greek.

My Greek grandparents on my father's side never accepted my mother because of her ethnicity. In the late sixties, many ethnic minorities—especially in New York—considered Puerto Ricans to be the lowest ethnic class. My Greek family believed my father married beneath him. Greeks married Greeks and, because they disapproved of the marriage, they disowned him. For a long time, our family was cut off from our Greek relatives and we only ever saw each other—at most—a couple of times a year.

Despite the challenges going into their relationship, they still married and started a family right away. They quickly had my brother, but then my mother suffered three miscarriages before she finally gave birth to me. My mother never felt like she had the support she needed from my father and it was the cause of many of their arguments. My parents had a rocky marriage from the beginning and they separated more times than I can count in their twenty-nine years together, but they never divorced.

One day, my mother packed up all her stuff and walked out of the apartment, leaving my brother and me behind. I believe she might have had a nervous breakdown and didn't know what else to do, so she left. At the time, I was only eleven and my brother wasn't much older. I begged my mother to come back, thinking it would be better if she did and I hoped that maybe things would be different. When she eventually moved back to Brooklyn, nothing changed with her drinking and life went back to the same roller coaster it had been before.

I kept the secret of my mother's alcoholism to myself for most of my childhood because I was embarrassed. Friends never came over; her drinking was too out in the open. We'd see my mother wake up in the morning, go to work, come home, pour a drink, and then pour another and another until she passed out. Talking about it wasn't an option. Even though things got bad, no one else in the family said anything to her. I knew this wasn't normal, but this was *my* normal.

Path to Wellness and Recovery

In high school, I made the decision to open up more to my close friends about what was going on at home. I worried about what they would say and how they might respond, but all I received from them was support and understanding. I learned that so many people I knew were also suffering in some way, some even with addiction and mental illness in their family. Now that I was talking more about things at home, some of the burden started to lift.

My answer to what was happening at home was to stay out of the house as much as possible. I started playing basketball at the Boys and Girls Club as an outlet. I began to change. I was becoming less destructive and confrontational and more focused. I went to school, basketball practice, and then home. For the first time, I started to build a support system and it started by sharing what was going on with my mom with a few close friends.

After my mother died, I struggled for a while. I drank almost every day for a year straight and was going down a dark path. It was a combination of things, including my faith in God, that pulled me out and got me through the pain of losing her. Somehow, the positive influences in my life helped keep me out of trouble. Those friends I opened up to back in high school are still friends today. I'm lucky I have them and, in many ways, they are some of the biggest supports I've ever known.

I consider myself lucky. There were so many directions I could have gone and negative forces in my life back then that I could have surrendered to. Three months after making the decision to clean up my act, I met my wife. Things moved fast—we got married and had our son in less than eighteen months. It may sound crazy, but I truly think my mother helped lead me to this exciting new life with my wife and family and for that I will be forever grateful to her.

Call to Action

My life has been a constant balance between two strong cultures. I have always tried to respect my Greek and Puerto Rican heritage, but know that both have traits and characteristics I want to protect my children from. I am lucky today to have my faith, a strong friend group, and my wife to support me, but I know others aren't as fortunate. So many young people today are growing up in multicultural and multiethnic households, like I did, where addiction and mental illness are prevalent. If my story can help them, I'm happy to share it.

For several years, I got into coaching youth basketball. I really felt I could make an impact that way. A big part of coaching is teaching kids how to become leaders, work together, and to support one another. Kids need to be taught coping skills and ways to manage difficult situations, and sports is a great way to learn this. Basketball was such an influential and positive outlet for me growing up that I found it natural to transition into coaching.

I spend my time today advocating for improved resources and supports for children and families. I know that mental health and addiction are hard to talk about, so I encourage people to have those difficult conversations. I urge parents to talk with their kids and tell them how having dinner together every night is a good place for these conversations to take place. There is power in being present. Not just physically there, but emotionally present, because kids see and appreciate that.

After going through a regional leadership program, I learned how Gracepoint—the largest behavioral health organization in the Tampa Bay area—helped thousands of children and adults each year with mental health and addiction challenges. I knew that I wanted to get involved and support those struggling in my community with a similar situation to mine. I joined the Gracepoint Foundation board of directors because it's important to me that I share my story and be a conduit to help others get the help they need.

The best decision I ever made was to start telling my story. I know, for many that can be hard, but when you are ready, I would encourage you to share it with the world. Above all, I encourage people to keep communicating, sharing awareness, and creating those safe spaces for conversation to happen.

Whether you are a caregiver, a concerned family member, or experiencing something yourself—I want you to know that you are not alone in this battle. Help is out there. It's never too late.

Jacquelyn Jamason

Licensed Mental Health Counselor

What I really want people to know is that we all have one thing in common, and that's resilience. No one sees the scars inside of us, so it's up to us to share what's there.

My Story

Six years…it has been six years since my phone buzzed on that remote beach island where I was kayaking with friends. Had I not looked down, I would not have even known the phone was ringing. On the other end, a woman was screaming, "Your baby is dead, Jacque! Dead! She killed her! Where are you?" This is when my life both ended as I knew it.

I screamed, dropped to my knees, and handed the phone to one of the other women. They pulled me up and, even though I felt myself moving and walking and talking, I don't remember any of it. The experience at the hospital was like something from a movie scene with police lining the halls and this strange quietness. I can't even begin to explain what happens when you see your daughter's lifeless dead body. I came home with my son that night but I had to leave Elliana behind—it was the worst experience of my life.

I've asked myself a thousand questions in the years since my daughter was murdered. How did I miss the signs? Why would anyone do this? I work in the mental health field and, even though I'm a trained licensed psychotherapist, I never saw any indications that led me to believe my former partner of more than 20 years would try to take our children's lives, then her own, I just didn't see it coming.

I had been in a codependent and unhealthy relationship for more than two decades. Kim was all I knew and all I had. When you are with a partner, with someone for that long, a strange familiarity seems to keep you stuck in place, like a hostage unable to leave. Even though the relationship was becoming more and more toxic all the time, I had become so codependent and reliant on her that I kept getting pulled back in. Our relationship was strained for several reasons—poor investments made worse by the recession of 2008 and Kim being against growing our family. She was addicted to sleeping pills and other narcotics, and the entire environment had become unhealthy.

I knew I needed an exit plan, but I still wanted her to be a part of the kids' lives. We talked about what separation would look like with us both living under the same roof, but I knew that was a bad idea.

My opportunity came while Kim was in a treatment center in Tennessee. I knew this was my time to get out because every time I had tried before, there was drama and it became impossible. I got out and moved into my own apartment; and, for the first time in as long as I could remember, I felt peaceful, free, and happy. I thought my life would finally start going in the direction I always wanted.

The truth about what happened that day is horrific. It was Kim's day to spend time with the kids. Kim had given the kids Xanax and she drowned Elli in the bathtub after my son fell asleep. My son woke up not feeling well, went looking for his little sister, and he used a knife to pry open the locked bathroom door. When he found Elli in the bathtub, he tried to resuscitate her but he couldn't. He called 911, but it was already too late. Elli died that day.

The first six months after it happened were the hardest. It was a high-profile murder case and we were trying to stay away from the media. My friends packed up my apartment; I never had to go back there again. We moved forty minutes north and thought we could start over. After only a month, I tried to go back to work. Not only was I not functioning, I was triggered constantly by my patients' stories of victimization and trauma.

> When a child dies - especially when the death is unexpected - surviving parents have a 67% higher risk of hospitalization for mental illness than do parents who never experience the death of a child.
>
> Source: MedPage Today

I was drinking all the time and having suicidal thoughts, not because I wanted to die but because I wanted a way to end my pain. It got to the point where I was putting a straw in the neck of a bottle of Fireball and drinking it as fast as I could. I found myself seeking relief for such disturbing thoughts by drinking, smoking, taking pills, excessive sleep, or just plain checking out. I knew that I may very well end my life if I didn't get the help I needed.

Although I had a son I needed to care for, it was all I could do to put my feet on the floor each morning and stumble into the living room. I compared it to sitting still while the world around me was zipping by at warp speed. I could hear people talking, asking me, '*How are you, are you eating, is there anything I can do*?' I didn't want to be "that" person. I didn't want to be the mom with a dead child, the mom of a murdered child. Day after day, waking up to my baby's little white cremation box with a pink bow on it, a large beautiful picture of her, and some of her prized possessions was becoming too much to bear.

Then I hit rock bottom. One day, I took my son to the skate park and was drinking in the car. I started drunk texting people. One of them was a friend who was in recovery herself. She came to the skate park, picked me up and took me directly to an AA meeting. A few days later, I went to a trauma-specific inpatient treatment facility for people who are dual diagnosed with addiction. I spent forty-five days there and it saved my life in so many ways.

Path to Wellness and Recovery

The treatment center was a dual diagnosis facility for mental health and addiction disorders that focused on individuals dealing with trauma, grief, and loss. I was forced to deal with everything that had happened.

The first week was terrible. I hated each and every minute of it. I wasn't an alcoholic. I wasn't as sick as "these people". I was there because my daughter was murdered and, after all, I was a licensed mental health counselor. I find that I'm now smirking at how my ego played out in those first weeks. I will never, ever, forget riding in the back of a "druggy buggy", the white van used to take all the clients to outside AA meetings or our big trip to Wal-Mart. At the time, I didn't understand how stripping me of all of my freedom then would give me so much freedom today. After I stopped fighting, I soon relished in not worrying about the outside world.

The Refuge became just that, a healing place for me. I found time to cry, write, breathe, talk, be silent, learn, paint, and to come to terms with my daughter's death and the cards I had been dealt. I felt tremendous guilt for not being with my son for such a long time, especially since I was missing his eleventh birthday, but I worked hard to remember that forty-five days is worth a lifetime if done well the first time.

About three weeks into treatment, I was told I couldn't graduate the program unless I worked on feeling and expressing anger as a component of grief. I was determined I was NOT going to lose control in this place in front of all these people. I was better than that! As usual, it took me a few days to process how I really felt. I was in my room one day and I began to fume over something small, like a sock being left on the floor. I ran as fast as I could to my therapist's cabin, asked for the baseball bat, and ran as fast as I could across campus to the tires where I could safely vent my anger. She yelled for me to wait, but I wasn't stopping. I went after those tires as if they were every single person who had ever hurt me in my life. I was yelling, screaming, and crying, until I couldn't stand anymore. I fell to the ground sobbing and just lay there. When I finally found the energy to stand, a group of my peers and my therapist were standing behind me, gently clapping and waiting to give me a hug. I felt as though I had finally allowed myself to start the healing process.

Although my healing was just beginning, it was time to go back into the real world, but I didn't leave alone. I met lifelong friends and supporters in sober men and women. I left with a newfound sense of life purpose, and the anti-depressants may have helped some, too. When I got home, I began regularly attending AA meetings. I didn't know if I was an alcoholic since I never really had any of the "problems" other alcoholics had in my life, but I knew if I wanted to live through this nightmare, I couldn't drink every time I felt the grief of losing Elliana.

Upon returning home, I was faced with attending court hearings for the first time since Elliana's murder. Because our case was high profile from the moment it happened, there were always news reporters present. I believe this is what may have saved me from doing anything stupid. Everything was being recorded—every breath, every move, *everything*. I had so much I wanted to say to the media, to the world, to Kim's family, yet I could not find the words.

For a year and a half, I didn't work. I took the time I needed to heal and grieve. I did therapy, went to yoga, and spent time with my son. After that, I got a job in a treatment center and started using my story as a platform to help other people. That honesty really catapulted me to the next level of healing, one where I was able to utilize my own journey as a way to have purpose and to start to walk my new normal.

In the beginning, I cried every day, all day. Then it was every other day. Then it was all I could do to get up and take a shower and brush my teeth or go to the store and not be triggered by everything, from a stroller to a baby crying. Grief really isn't linear; it's messy and it's all over the place, and I'm continually trying to find ways to work through my feelings as they change over the years.

There are still days when I simply can't do today. I take a day off, and work through the self-care that I need, then I dig back in. For a long time, I didn't plan out the next day, week, or month. I have adapted more and more as time goes on. It's true what they say—it just takes time.

From day one at the hospital, I have been blessed enough to have had the loving support of my church family, friends, immediate family, and the community as a whole. Each court appearance was jam-packed with supporters and advocates for my son and me. We were held up each and every day by other people and even sometimes anonymous angels.

My self-care regimen has included many things; fitness, education, and professional development. The one that has impacted me the most is how I have embraced fitness and training into my everyday life. In 2017, I was introduced to the SMART Ride (Southern Most AIDS/HIV Ride), a bike ride starting in Miami and ending in Key West. The ride totaled five hundred riders, raising money for AIDS awareness. It started at the University of Miami and ended on the beach in Key West.

Those two days, and a hundred and sixty-five miles, changed my life.

> Alcoholism is a very serious problem in the LGBTQ community. Up to 25 percent of the general LGBTQ community has moderate alcohol dependency, compared to 5 to 10 percent of the general population.
>
> Source: Alcohol Rehab Guide

I didn't know what I was doing. The physical toll it took on my body was a metaphor for life. At the end I realized: If I can do this, I can do life. The psychological benefits of fitness have been huge in my healing. My calendar is filled now with a run this day, a bike ride that day, and in 2019 I competed in my first triathlon. I love the joy of competition, testing my limits, and the camaraderie with people who have also suffered and been through some real personal struggles.

Focusing on the here and now, being right where my feet are and not getting stuck in what's behind or ahead of me, has really helped me. It wasn't until the five-year mark that I trusted life enough to even plan ahead more than a day at a time, then a week, then a month, and now the year for vacations, birthdays, anniversaries, etc.

Although I have had many slips, relapses, or recurring drinking episodes, I am now celebrating three years of sobriety. Everything I have learned about dealing with life on life's terms is from the twelve-step program of Alcoholics Anonymous. I have learned that there will be days when I wake up and don't want to face life, want to die, or my teenage son has decided to be my arch nemesis; but now I have tools to work through whatever life throws at me.

I worry all the time about my son. I've already lost one child, and I sometimes have anxiety and panic about what I'll find when I get home. I know I can't always be there to protect him. Being in a recovery program has taught me to detach with love, to give him the tools he needs, and to keep having those conversations. He thanks me all the time for talking with him and listening to what he's going through.

Though much has transpired in my personal and professional life since 2014, the most healing has occurred this past year as my son and I have been finally able to have conversations with one another that are hard and powerful. There is plenty of unresolved residual anger, but we have chosen to move through this life's storms together and intact.

Call to Action

I'm ready to talk. We need to draw attention to addiction, to domestic violence in same-sex relationships, to trauma and what it can do to you. My friends are no longer afraid to ask me how I'm doing and I'm not afraid to tell them the truth.

That's what I want to do—talk about Elli's story and keep her memory alive. Elli was a free spirit who was always telling jokes and laughing. She lived every single moment to the fullest, and that's how I'm trying to live now. I want to tell people, "Don't waste a single moment. Take the pictures, film the videos, go on the adventures. Don't take any of it for granted."

I've been asked to speak at local events on domestic violence awareness days. These are helpful because they incite a sense of power for my voice in these discussions. There is always the fear that the carpet will be ripped out from under you and, at times, it's visceral. Speaking out for the cause takes a certain level of authenticity and vulnerability, and that is scary.

What I really want people to know is that we all have one thing in common, and that's resilience. Once you've been through a traumatic experience, you have two choices: Give up and give in or find some purpose and meaning in what happened and hope your story helps someone else. I've chosen to see the purpose and meaning.

No one sees the scars inside of us, so it is up to us to share what's there.

Ian M. Adair

Nonprofit Executive /
Speaker and Author

*Mental illness and substance abuse destroyed my family.
Watching and caring for loved ones battle these diseases
shaped my life. Now I have an opportunity and the
platform to change the conversation around mental
health from one that condemns and diminishes those
suffering, to one of empathy and support.*

My Story

I got home late, just after 11:00 p.m., and immediately noticed there was no one there. This was strange because my mother had been battling cancer for months and rarely left the house. When she finally got home a few minutes after me, I could tell something was really wrong and that she was upset. She wasted no time telling me that my older brother had tried to kill himself, the university staff had found him just in time, and that he was in the hospital. My world, in that one moment, completely fell apart.

Just getting home that night from a long weekend in Texas was an adventure in itself. I remember the date—Sunday, November 8th, 1992— because I was out of town to watch my prep school play our championship football game and check out a university near Dallas for myself while visiting a friend. Neither of the experiences went very well, and by early Sunday evening I was back on I-35, heading home to Oklahoma City.

If anything, the ride home was the most exciting part of the trip. Mainly because I fell asleep at the wheel and drove a short distance between both sides of the highway through a rocky median. A jolt from going over a rock, which caused me to hit my head on the roof of my car, woke me up and I quickly pulled over to the side of the road in a panic. Someone even pulled over to check on me and said they were behind me honking for some time in horror of what might happen. I remember thinking how stupid I was and the guilt that came over me for being so reckless with my life, I knew my mom would be upset when I told her. I never got a chance to share that story with her.

I really don't remember much that happened in any detail over the weeks and months that followed. The shock of the news seemed to paralyze me and left me numb to most things that would have normally bothered me at school or with my friends. The emptiness I walked around with had to be noticeable to the people in my life, but no one said anything. I know there were hospital visits, counseling sessions, long emotional discussions, and sleepless nights, but time seemed to just pass by.

It was my senior year of high school, that time in my life was mostly spent taking care of my mother who was undergoing cancer treatment and doing everything I could to keep what our family was going through a secret from the world. No one really knew that much about us. To us, the truth would be used against us in some way. So my father's drug problem, how he abandoned us, the constant moving from city to city, living on government assistance—and, of course, the mental illness—was all kept a secret most of my life.

At one point, I was even living alone because Mom had been admitted to the hospital for her cancer treatment immediately after my brother was hospitalized. I was on a support list at my school and individuals or families would bring over food, almost every day. The gesture was nice, but the frequency I actually found inconvenient and disruptive; I just wanted to be left alone. Someone must have thought my situation was odd because a social worker and police officer came by one day to check on me because they thought it as reported I was a minor living alone. It was explained to me that this was a neglect investigation case and they wanted to come in and ask me some questions. For the first time, being held back in the ninth grade was about to pay off because I was already eighteen years old. The police officer looked at my driver's license and said there was nothing they could do, I was an adult, and he wished me well and left the house. I don't recall what I actually said to the social worker, but I know it was not very nice because I remember he walked away frustrated and shaking his head.

> Only about one-third of those suffering from an anxiety disorder receive treatment, even though the disorders are highly treatable.
>
> Source: Anxiety and Depression Association of America

Looking back on that day, there were signs that eventually led to my brother thinking suicide was his only way out. The biggest was after I received a call from my father on Tuesday, November 3rd—the day is easy to remember because it is my father's birthday. The call was completely random—we had no contact with him for a few years at that point—it had no significance in terms of substance, but I told my brother about it anyway. He was really upset about me even taking the call and grilled me for a long time about what was said and how things were left. I tried to reassure him it was our absent jackass of a dad just being himself, completely unaware of the reality and still unwilling to pay child support or support us in any way, but things for my brother seemed to spiral out of control from there and his suicide attempt was a few days later.

> According to the latest available data 494,169 people visited a hospital for injuries due to self-harm, suggesting that approximately 12 people harm themselves for every reported death by suicide.
>
> Source: American Foundation for Suicide Prevention

When I was finally allowed to visit my brother in the hospital, all he could ever say to me was, "I'm not crazy." He never discussed his suicide attempt with me, not once, and did his best over the following years to forget or acknowledge it ever happened. My mother became incredibly focused on my brother's emotional state and we never discussed the attempt; we were all in denial. Looking back on this time, I still feel a deep sadness. With each year after high school, I grew further apart from my mother and brother. Even though we had lived through so much together, there just was not much connecting our family anymore.

My father was gone, my mother and brother had their own codependent life together, and I was alone. It was soon after I finished college that I first started feeling real symptoms of depression. For me, these included constant exhaustion and fatigue, I was restless and had trouble sitting still, and feeling empty most of the day. I suffered from insomnia off and on for years, but things were getting worse and it was becoming increasingly difficult to sleep. I also was not finding any joy in things I had loved for a long time and, after a lifetime of playing tennis at both the college and professional level, I gave up the sport.

These feelings stayed with me for a couple of years and then evolved into something stronger. I suffered my first anxiety attack when I was twenty-five years old and it scared the hell out of me. I felt like my heart was pounding out of my chest and, even though I just came out of the shower, I started sweating and felt incredibly lightheaded. I must have slid down the wall in the bathroom because I remember becoming alert again a few minutes later, still in a towel sitting on the ground, and wondering what just happened. The attacks continued for the next couple of years, but I was lucky—they were not consistent or frequent and I was usually at home alone when they occurred. I feared going out in public in case an attack might happen. I knew I needed to address this soon, but the stigma in those days was very unforgiving. You were either healthy or labeled crazy, there was little in between.

Most of my twenties were filled with excuses for why my depression and anxiety kept me away from friends, events, and celebrations I was expected to attend. I struggled with insomnia, months at a time, for close to ten years. My eating habits were all over the place and my weight constantly fluctuated, but the most unexpected symptom was that I always seemed to be in pain and suffered from headaches, daily. I had recovered from a couple of bad car accidents and some injuries from playing sports, the physical symptoms from my mental illness really started to bother me, especially the severe back pain I was experiencing.

Even though we had been through so much as a family, I knew I could not go to them because of how badly our relationship had deteriorated. It had gotten so bad that now we went long stretches of time without communicating, sometimes going longer than a year without talking. In reality we were all suffering, but at the time we could not see it that clearly. Though we all had a shared experience together, we were fixated on keeping our separate experiences and our pain from each other. We became more distant, so every time I got the opportunity to move away from them—usually across the country—I took it.

Telling my own story was never really an option for me while my mother was still alive because I ranked her pain and suffering, both mentally and physically, over mine. She lived a hard life, at the time she had enough to worry about, and I did not want to add to that. I felt that if I shared what I was going through it would somehow diminish her suffering. A completely foolish thought, I know; but, when you think about it, we all do it. When someone we love has suffered a trauma or is going through a really bad situation, we keep our own problems to ourselves, especially if we feel they are suffering more.

Path to Wellness and Recovery

I think most people who have mental illness in their family seek to discover more about their family's medical history and learn more about those who suffered. I was no different, probably explaining why all of my degrees and certifications are in behavioral science. I knew, from all of my formal education, that I was not alone and that I could get help. It still took a lot for me to finally talk with someone and figure out what worked best for me to manage my mental health, but the work I finally put in was worth it because it got me to where I am today.

After reconnecting with my mother's side of the family several years after she passed away, I learned even more about her struggle with mental illness and a suicide attempt she never told me about. For years, I witnessed mental health and addiction in my family, but it took me a while to come to grips with my own. We all experience mental illness differently. Too many self-medicate, ignore the signs and symptoms, or fear they are alone in their suffering. After you identify an issue, the real challenge comes in how you are going to respond to it.

I knew that, in order to heal, I had to start forgiving myself for thinking I could have done more to help those around me who had suffered or died. My brother's suicide attempt was something I could not stop. My mother's every day battle with mental illness was something I could not fix. My closest friend in college died after a long battle with addiction, and I carried around a lot of guilt for a long time believing I could have done more to help him. Recovery and healing really have so much to do with forgiveness. Forgiving others can be hard but forgiving yourself can sometimes feel impossible.

My path to wellness has been paved with small successes, teachable moments, and daily affirmations. Sometimes even the little things, like getting out of bed and eating, can be difficult. So I start every day with one simple action—making my bed. I read it somewhere that even the smallest victory or success early in your day can help propel you to keep moving forward. So that's what I did, I forced myself out of bed and then made it. I consider this to be the best advice I ever learned concerning managing my mental health, and continue the practice to this day.

Taking care of yourself is hard work—actually, it's really hard work—and managing mental illness is an everyday and forever process. You constantly have to value your accomplishments more than anyone else and block out anyone trying to diminish you. You have to let yourself know you are doing a great job and, most importantly, you have to be proud of your work and efforts.

My self-care involved addressing some real factors impacting my mental health. I had to remove people from my life who were draining me both mentally and emotionally. That included family and longtime close friends. I'm open to welcoming people back, but you have to recognize that recovery requires the right support system and people to help bring out the best in you. Every major accomplishment in my life has happened after I went through this process and, although I miss having certain people around at times, I know I made the best decision for me.

Call to Action

Around the age of forty, I really started to open up more about my family's challenges with mental health and addiction. The more I shared, the more liberating those moments became, and I felt free for the first time. Everything became clearer in my mind—not just what I no longer feared in my life, but what I wanted from it.

I ultimately became a mental health advocate for a lot of reasons, some are deeply personal and others I'm more open about. My goal with every presentation, article I write, and speech I give is to end the stigma associated with mental illness and addiction so those suffering get the help they need. Fear should not keep someone from getting treatment or help, but that is the power stigma has over us.

As an advocate for mental health awareness, my mission is clear: mental illness and substance abuse destroyed my family. Watching and caring for loved ones who battle these diseases shaped my life. Now I have an opportunity and the platform to change the conversation around mental health from one that condemns and diminishes those suffering to one of empathy and support.

Every chance I get, I remind people that we all go through painful situations and fight battles many will never know. To everyone working on managing their recovery or mental illness: I want you to know that you are strong, you will get through this. And when you do, be proud of your resilience and progress, every day. I was silent about my depression for so long and kept what I was going through hidden from everyone in my life, even close family and friends. It can take a while until you feel comfortable to share your story, but now that I am there—I never want to be silent again. I want anyone suffering to know—help is out there; you are never alone.

I encourage everyone to speak their truth. Remember that humility, vulnerability and authenticity go a long way in reaching your audience. You never know who your story will inspire, motivate, or even save—so keep sharing it!

Vanessa McNeal

Documentary Film Maker / Executive Director, Story Maven Media

The highest form of healing, for me, continues to be gratitude. I am grateful for what I have gone through because it has molded me into the woman I am today. It has taught me about what it means to forgive, love, and choose your own fate, even after you feel like it's already been chosen for you.

My Story

When I was three or four years old, my sister and I were sent down to the basement because the adults were hosting a party upstairs. We were down there playing Barbies under the pool table when my older cousin came by and asked us if we wanted to have sex. I had no idea what the word *sex* meant or what was about to happen. She proceeded to molest my sister and me, one by one, in front of each other. She then forced my sister to molest me in front of her. Soon thereafter, my sister chose to molest me without my cousin's orders, almost every day for several years.

At the age of fifteen, I was sexually assaulted by an older boy while I was away from home attending a summer college prep program. In the lawsuit with the college that followed, I was forced to overcome the many faces of rape culture, specifically the shaming and silence that usually surrounds sexual assault victims. I was diagnosed with PTSD and suffered from anxiety and depression. At seventeen, I attempted suicide.

People have to know that sexual violence, no matter the severity or type, is a guilt- and shame-inducing experience. It changes who you are; it changes almost everything about you. For so much of my life, I struggled with trusting people and with feeling safe in my own body. My worldview was completely altered by what happened to me. I never told anyone; I never even felt like telling was an option. My voice, my innocence, and my power of choice was ripped away from me—at a very early age.

I loved school and was the first person in my family to graduate from high school as well as the first

> 94% of women who are raped experience symptoms of post-traumatic stress disorder (PTSD) during the two weeks following the rape.
>
> Source: RAINN (Rape, Abuse & Incest National Network)

to go to college. I got a full ride scholarship to Iowa State University and, when I got there, I was able to finally see a different world. College gave me the opportunity to see life through a different lens.

I enrolled in a human sexuality class my freshman year at ISU. My professor took the time to define sexual violence. She also defined molestation. She followed these definitions by bravely and unapologetically sharing her personal story of being a survivor of sexual violence. My professor stood in front of our class, with no shame, and owned her experience. She wasn't a victim, she was a survivor—and I wanted to be that, too. That moment gave me power and totally changed my life.

This was the first time in my life I had a name for my own experience. I always thought I was the only one who had experienced these violent acts. Until that moment, I had never heard someone else's story before. Her bravery and strength inspired me. In that moment, I didn't know who I was but I knew who I could be. I could be a victor instead of a victim. I could be strong and powerful, like her.

She was the first person I shared my story with and she filled me with hope and reassurance, assuring me there was a life outside the world I knew. She let me know I could find a life of healing and, when I found that, I would find my voice. She gave me the confidence to own my story and stand powerfully in my experience. That's when I started the work of healing.

Path to Wellness and Recovery

In college, it doesn't seem to be as taboo to go to therapy as it is in the professional world. I enrolled in a trauma therapy group on campus. This group of survivors created a community of women who had experienced similar trauma. There was so much shared power in that group. It helped us all realize that we were not alone and we supported one another through our different journeys.

I spent my college years healing and growing. Then, one night, a friend asked me, "What do you want your legacy to be?" No one had asked me that question before. The seed was planted and I went home inspired. I already knew my legacy would be driven by my desire to share my personal story with anyone and everyone I could.

I got into film during my senior year of college. Film is such a powerful form of storytelling. The realization that I could share my story in documentary form took hold and I started reaching out to local filmmakers. Because of my professor's honesty, I had the courage to research and write a documentary about my own life. I talked about my experiences with sexual violence and, even though it was the hardest thing I ever had to do, it changed my life and allowed me to impact the lives of many others.

After sharing my own story, I realized that I was part of a community that was so big I really couldn't even wrap my head around it. I think a lot of people worry that no one will care if you share your story, but there are so many people who do care and even more willing to support you along the way.

Recovery is hard and you have to put in the work. I believe we have really wronged each other as far as our expectations concerning healing. We have been taught that an incident happens, we work on it, and then there's a resolution to it. We talk about trauma like it has a start and end point, but that's not how trauma works. Healing is not linear. There are times when you have to forgive someone over and over again, just as there are times you have to forgive yourself over and over again.

The practice of self-care is so important in my life and plays a large role in my healing. I meditate, pray, get massages, and spend time in nature. Still, to this day, I am in therapy and see it as needed maintenance. Having a nonjudgmental person who can listen to me helps me process my fears, beliefs, and everyday challenges. Self-care is even when I decide not to do anything for a whole day and I don't have any guilt about it because I'm using that time to nourish my soul. When I finally understood how connected my mind/body/soul were, I was able to find techniques that nurtured all three.

The highest form of healing for me continues to be gratitude. I am grateful for what I have gone through because it has molded me into the woman I am today. It taught me what it means to forgive, love, and choose your own fate—even after you feel like it's already been chosen for you.

I am always processing my trauma and learning about how it impacts my life, even today. I wake up every day knowing I will spend the rest of my life healing and that my healing is forever. The experience of enduring sexual violence will not go away, but knowing you aren't alone helps to tame the trauma. You have an opportunity to change the narrative of your life if you want to—that's up to you, not anyone else.

Call to Action

One of the most rewarding ways I have shared my story and the story of others is through the documentary films I produce and direct. Through sharing these stories, I have educated the public, created a community for survivors, and inspired legislators to improve policies for crime victims. My purpose is to help heal the hurt, give company to the alone, and give hope to those in despair who feel there is no way out. I want to inspire other people to take ownership of their story and not be afraid or ashamed of it.

Your story is part of the relationship of who you are, who you can become, and who you can grow to be in the outside world. Stories have the power to break the chains of oppression and bring about healing. More importantly, stories also have the power to release others from their own silence.

After my documentary aired about my experience, eight individuals reached out to me and let me know they too were sexual abuse survivors. I saw there was a need for more people to speak out and share what happened to them. To give those eight people a platform and voice, I created my next film, *We Are Survivors,* in 2015. Almost every person I have worked with saw their self-confidence boosted dramatically because they were able to talk about what happened to them. They were no longer alone and they felt heard. Sexual violence affects one in four women and one in six men. For the people who have watched the film, there was an overwhelming shock because they didn't realize how common sexual violence is.

From the research and feedback I received after *We Are Survivors,* I decided my next project would address male sexual violence. I directed *The Voiceless,* an award-winning documentary about five male survivors of sexual violence. There is so much more social stigma on men who are sexually abused and even less empathy and support for men who do share when sexual violence happens to them. When I made the documentary, I found it very interesting that all of the men we worked with had different stories but they shared a common thread—they didn't feel like men. We've created a world where if you don't meet certain criteria, then you're not a man; and that's not right.

My latest film, *Gridshock,* is an investigative documentary exposing the hidden and disturbing reality behind the sex trafficking demand in Iowa. This documentary shines a light on buyers of sex-trafficked women and how they fuel the demand for further exploitation. The film seeks to learn who the buyers are and why there is a culture of impunity where they are concerned. In search of these answers, I interview survivors, local and federal law enforcement, politicians, and a recovering sex addict.

Outside of being a filmmaker, I am a national speaker. I share my story at colleges/universities, conferences, and at special events. I founded Story Maven Media, a nonprofit organization elevating social issues through film. Being able to unapologetically share your life and your story with the world gives you a huge sense of freedom. That's the power of story.

> 1 out of every 6 American women has been the victim of an attempted or completed rape in her lifetime.
>
> Source: RAINN (Rape, Abuse & Incest National Network)

When I look at my life and what I have done with it, I see the purpose in my pain. I do not have anger or resentment for my trauma anymore. I know now that it wasn't all for nothing. We all need to realize that we're more alike than we are different and we share so many similar experiences.

I don't know where I'd be without my professor's story. She changed everything and, for me, what I am doing is redemption for the little girl in me that I honor. It gives what I went through a purpose and meaning, along with the knowledge that none of it was in vain and that I can do something that makes the world a better place because of it.

I'm not a victim any more. I am a survivor. You are not what happened to you, you are what you chose to become. Speaking up and discussing sexual violence is really hard, but necessary work. I know I'm exactly where I'm supposed to be when I'm speaking. I want everyone to know that it gets better. Over time, you will be thankful for the growth you were able to make and the resiliency you were able to find.

Several people took things from me without my permission so, every day, I'm fighting to take that back for myself. Although I have had many challenges in my life, I survived them, overcame them, and I want people to know they can, too. You're not alone.

Ray Sikorski

CEO & President, Verified Label, Print & Promotions

I want people to know that mental illness is a treatable condition. I want to encourage those who are suffering to just take that first step and, with each step forward, let them know the next one gets easier.

My Story

It was 4:00 a.m. on Saturday morning when the phone rang. I rolled over, checked my phone, and saw it was my parents calling, not a good sign. I didn't answer it. I got up, went into the bathroom, splashed some water on my face, and just stared at my reflection in the mirror. I said to myself, *I bet Jimmy's dead.* If he was just in the hospital again, my parents would have waited a few more hours before calling me. I gathered my thoughts for a moment, then called them back and I was right, my youngest brother had killed himself.

My dad, as calm as a man talking about a fender-bender he'd had last week, gave me the details of what happened. Two police officers had come by their house and woke them up around 1:30 a.m. Jim was living with his girlfriend. They'd gone to bed around 10:00 p.m. and she heard a loud noise around 10:30 p.m. Jim had gotten up, gone into the bathroom, and shot himself with a handgun he'd picked up earlier that week. From the way Jim lay on the bathroom floor, they thought he probably watched himself do it in the mirror, so it appeared to be intentional. Their place became a crime scene and standard procedures were followed; they questioned his girlfriend, and tested her fingers for gun powder, and ruled it a suicide.

As my dad shared the story the police officers told him, his voice cracked, he paused, and then he started to cry. After a moment, he told me, "It didn't seem real, until I hear myself telling it to you. And now I can't believe it. I can't believe he's gone." It was October 16th, and we were just about to start the worst holiday season of our lives.

We were a tight-knit family, had a great upbringing, and loving parents. I was the oldest of us three boys, Steve is three years younger than me, and Jimmy was six years younger. Despite our age difference, Jim and I had a lot of similar interests and, for much of my life, he was one of my closest friends in addition to being my little brother. That became the hardest part for me, the feeling that I didn't do my job as a big brother. I spent a lot of time beating myself up, wishing I had done more. Despite how close we all were, none of us could stop what happened.

Jim was a licensed mental health counselor and worked in the mental health and substance abuse field for fifteen years. He'd run group therapy sessions, family sessions, worked with adults, and also worked with kids. With his professional background, Jimmy knew he needed help but didn't want the stigma of being a mental health patient. He wouldn't commit to the treatment. He often explained the downward mental health progression, through feeling helpless to hopeless to worthless, and how he had started feeling those same things about himself. He had built up so much negative momentum that he couldn't break out of it. We told him many times how much he was loved, but he just couldn't see how we felt anymore. His depression got the better of him and he tried to escape those feelings with drugs and alcohol.

About 6% of American adults (about 15 million people) have an alcohol use disorder, but only about 7% of Americans who are addicted to alcohol ever receive treatment.

Source: Addiction Center

Because of his training and education, Jim knew what was happening to him and where he was headed if it didn't stop. He knew our family's history with mental illness and recognized the symptoms when they started to show themselves in his life. He had an increasing problem with depression and a growing feeling of paranoia. He was using drugs and alcohol, at first for fun but increasingly more as an escape.

As he got older, his addiction started impacting his life in significant ways. He lost three or four mental health jobs over the years after going on benders and disappearing from work a week at a time. We would find him after the worst of these occurrences, passed out on the floor of his townhouse surrounded by sixty or more empty wine and liquor bottles. These occasions would usually land him in the hospital for a few days. The first couple times, this really scared the hell out of us as a family. But by the third time, I was starting to understand that no one drinks that much unless they're trying to kill themselves.

No matter how much we all pushed, Jim always resisted ongoing treatment or twelve-step programs like AA. He knew he would lose his license to practice in the mental health field if the depth of his problems became known. He didn't want the help of the family and pulled away from us more and more. There was so much he needed to admit, to others, and most of all to himself. But he could never be honest with himself, or with his family, because he was so ashamed of his choices and the person he felt he'd become. What he never realized—and what breaks my heart—is that we would have loved him all the more if he had admitted his struggles and opened up to us.

Within months after my brother's death, I started to see a steady decline in my own physical and mental health. I was crying all the time, depressed, experiencing headaches, and my eyesight was worsening. Our family has a history of high blood pressure and heart problems, so seeing my family doctor for a physical was a mandatory yearly event. If it's possible to fail a physical, I did—and miserably. My weight and blood pressure were up, my cholesterol was high, and my liver and kidney numbers were going in the wrong direction. Overall, it was the worst single-year drop in my health that I'd ever had, and I wasn't surprised.

On top of all of my health problems, I was drinking a lot more than usual. A growing number of people close to me had also noticed and pointed this out to me. So far, they were pretty much giving me a pass on my drinking because of my brother's suicide. Also, because I was an easy, good-natured drinker, no one saw my behavior as self-destructive. My doctor, however, would not give me a pass and confronted me about my health, and what would happen if I didn't start to make some changes. I knew it was time to pull my head out of my ass.

I'd tried halfheartedly, several times, to get over my brother's death and get back to some kind of normal. Get back to working full time, stop being sad, and cut back on my drinking, but it hadn't worked. I'd gone through a pretty rough divorce a few years earlier, and it had taught me a process. Moving on with my life would require some small positive decisions and commitments, leading to bigger ones, and so on. It was a conscious decision-making process, not something that just happens one day. It was time to get to work.

Path to Wellness and Recovery

A couple weeks after Jimmy's death, partly at my urging, mom and dad had gone to a series of Al-Anon meetings. This is where families and friends of alcoholics and drug users get together to talk about their experiences and help each other try to recover. It worked miracles for my parents, helping them to realize that Jimmy's suicide was not their fault. Although they eventually stopped going, my mom was still looking for some additional support, because she was struggling hard with Jimmy's death. I really wanted to help her and be there for her, but I wasn't doing much better at that time.

I've always been one of those people who talks to himself, but lately I'd been talking to Jimmy. I'd been telling him how much I missed him and how much I wish he had reached out for help during those last days. So, as step one in my official improvement plan, I started writing down what I wanted to say. That process really helped.

I'd learned from a business speaker years earlier that your mind replays things over and over to help you remember them. So these thoughts take up space in the forefront of your mind and clouds your focus on the other current events around you. But when you write things down, it gives your brain permission to move on and stop trying to remember those thoughts.

Six months after Jimmy passed away, the writing was helping me put his death into perspective. It worked so well, I progressed to writing a brief history of all the significant events of my life. I'd had a lot of good events, some with all my family and others with my brothers, Jimmy and Steve, but a lot of them were on my own or with other people. So, I began to see that my life would go on and it would continue to be full.

I also started reaching out to other people whom I'd learn had been through similar losses. Suicide is uncomfortably common and it turns out I know at least a dozen people who have been through the loss of someone close to them. Hearing their stories, and sharing mine with them, was tremendously cathartic. I even wrote some of them down so I could remind myself that this is unfortunately part of life.

I joined a gym and started working out four or five mornings a week. I'd always exercised and stayed in reasonable shape, but it was time to kick it up a notch. Consistent strenuous exercise builds positive momentum in many ways and, for me, it's the most effective way to fight back negative thoughts and feelings. Fairly quickly, I started feeling a little better. Then I started eating a little better, drinking a little less, going to bed a little earlier, and it snowballed from there. As long as I was getting up early and making it to the gym, then I felt like I was pointed in the right direction and making progress.

Things were finally moving in the right direction for me and I was looking forward to seeing my family more often. I'd cut back on them because being around them reminded me of Jimmy so much and brought about so many sad feelings. I noticed, after a while, that I could think and talk about Jimmy without feeling down or sad. That was important, especially for my mom. She was the most affected by Jimmy's death and she needed us around more often. She needed to talk about it and I found that I could now do that with her.

> A loss due to suicide can be among the most difficult losses to bear and may leave the survivors with a tremendous burden of guilt, anger and shame. Survivors may even feel responsible for the death.
>
> Source: Mental Health America

Losing Jim has left a permanent hole in our family. We have chosen to focus on his birthday each year instead of the day he died, celebrating the life he gave to this world and the memories we have of this smart, amazing man.

I've learned two important things through all this. One, how hard it can be to forgive yourself for not doing or saying more. Two, the person who is struggling is the one who has to make the decision to get treatment, otherwise it will never last. You can't save someone who's not ready to be saved. You can't make someone behave the way you want them to. You can't force someone get therapy, take medication, or stop drinking. We've all heard this before, but you can't understand how true it is until you've lived it.

Call to Action

The saddest part about my brother's death is that he knew mental illness and substance abuse are often co-existing conditions, and they are treatable. The more we learn about how the brain works, the more we understand that it's a physical process. He knew where his addiction and mental illness would take him if he did not get help. So, I now make it my personal mission to make others aware that help is out there, and life can get better if they make the effort.

I'm an active board member at Gracepoint, one of the largest behavioral health organizations in Florida. I have actually served on three different boards within the organization and currently sit on two. Although I was involved with Gracepoint before my brother's death, I knew it was something I had to reengage with and get back in my life. My involvement with them makes me feel good about myself, and I know that I'm making a difference and supporting people who need help.

As an advocate for mental health and addiction services, I see the obstacles facing those who suffer. Until we start seeing mental health disorders as a treatable condition, the shame and stigma will always be there for people like my brother. People don't feel ashamed of needing insulin to treat their diabetes and they shouldn't feel ashamed of needing treatment for their mental illness or addiction.

Things are changing in society, mostly for the better, but not fast enough on mental health. We need to look at mental illness as a physical disease, like cancer or the high blood pressure I inherited from my father. Research is now showing that those who have a family history of mental illness have a higher risk of developing an issue.

Too many of us are too afraid of the unknown, so we stay in places that we know are terrible and toxic for us. I want people to know that mental illness is a treatable condition. I want to encourage those who are suffering to just take that first step and, with each step forward, let them know the next one gets easier.

I know I'll never be fully healed because my life forever changed when Jim died. I miss him. I celebrate him. And now I share his story to help others. If you are suffering, you have nothing to be ashamed of. Please seek help. Lean on your loved ones; you are never alone.

Bill Lutes

Bank Market President for Tampa Bay & Southwest Florida

Healing is ultimately about the survivors, not the lost.
My grief was like a shoebox in a closet that I opened
every day, then it became every other day, which turned
into once a week, and now I open it only when I need to.

My Story

Andrew's room was the apartment over the garage. I opened the door, called his name, and got no response. I walked up the stairs, called his name again, and still…nothing. I noticed that the light in the bathroom was still on. I saw that his bed was unmade and his bag was sitting on the floor. From where I was standing, I could see his body in the bathtub. I knew. That awful, sickening feeling in the pit of my stomach that told me it was already too late. I screamed over and over again, "Andrew's dead! Andrew's dead!"

To this day, I remember every detail about how I found my son. Andrew's right hand hanging out of the bathtub, the tilt of his head, where blood was splattered, and the gun on his body. I ran down to tell my wife Paula, who had heard my screams. She told her parents who were visiting that day, to get our youngest son, Will, out of the house, while she called 911.

Everything after finding my son that January 7th evening, is a giant blur. The time I spent with the coroner, watching police seal my son's room as a crime scene, talking with investigators, the visit from our priest (who I questioned if this suicide meant Andrew would still go to heaven), and even seeing those who had been in the house that day that had to come back for questioning—since this was technically a crime scene, until ruled otherwise.

Andrew's future seemed so bright. He had just graduated with honors from the University of Florida, had been recruited by the big four accounting firms, and he had already accepted an internship with one in Atlanta. Then, in an instant, it was over.

There was no note, nothing at all to tell us what he was thinking in those final moments. He didn't call his older brother or his mother, his girlfriend, or roommates at college, or reach out to anyone to tell them he was depressed, suffering, or suicidal. For a long time, it was easy to judge and blame myself for not noticing something, anything. I was his father, after all—how did I miss this?

All I could do for months in my grief and despair was search for answers. Why? Why would he do this? Why wouldn't he have talked to us? To anyone? I spoke to everyone he knew—roommates, recruiters, advisors, professors, the dean, and they were all as bewildered as our family. No one saw this coming. No one saw Andrew, someone who had never shot a gun in his life, as a young man who would take my gun and end his life.

The morning before he died, he paid his share of the utility bills for the rental house he shared with his friends from school. Then, an hour or two later, he shot himself. For a while, I struggled to understand how a person could go from thinking rationally to thinking so irrationally. How could Andrew take a temporary problem and resolve it with a permanent solution?

The truth is there were signs of depression long before that night. Things that he was experiencing that we didn't recognize until we looked back. His friends had noticed he was more withdrawn and stayed in his room more instead of socializing. He was dealing with insomnia and his inability to sleep had become so intolerable that he was smoking marijuana to help him. He was less responsive to text messages and phone calls. He wasn't shaving every day, started wearing the same shirts over and over again, and became less concerned about his appearance. For a meticulous kid like Andrew, this was unusual behavior.

My thoughts always take me back to the night before Andrew took his life. Nothing happened that evening that seemed different than any other night. We sat in the living room watching the Florida State University national championship game. We laughed and talked, discussing whether Auburn running back Tre Mason could have changed the outcome of the game and where he was projected to be in the NFL. When the game was over, Andrew said he was heading back to school in the morning

> The suicide rate among American men is about four times higher than among women, according to data from the Centers for Disease Control and Prevention.
>
> Source: American Psychological Association

and promised to let me know when he arrived. Before heading to his room, he told me he loved me and gave me a hug.

Andrew, like so many others who die by suicide, learned to mask his pain and suffering. He put on a big smile, was loving and caring, and was always willing to help and please others. I tried to understand what led him to this decision, but the more I learned about severe depression, the more I came to understand that Andrew was simply a young man struggling with an undiagnosed mental health condition. The reality was he was hurting badly, nobody knew how much, and he saw no other way out.

Path to Wellness and Recovery

Andrew and I were very close and my world was rocked. I knew my life would never be the same. The death of a child is one of the most traumatic things anyone can go through. Losing a child to suicide is the ultimate trauma for a parent, something I realized in the weeks and months after his death. No one grieves the same and we all deal with grief and loss differently. While no one ever totally recovers from the loss of a loved one, over time you get to a point where the pain becomes manageable.

I very quickly learned that losing a child to suicide also made me a member of an exclusive club that no one wants to be a part of. Still, I was fortunate to have the opportunity to speak with several other parents who also lost a child to suicide. I found they were the only people that truly understood the depth of my loss and pain.

Getting back to normal seemed impossible. As a family, we tried suggestions and ideas from anyone and everyone. We tried remodeling the garage apartment where Andrew died, but it didn't help, so we ended up moving. We tried to make the anniversary of Andrew's death a day focused on celebrating his life, but it was difficult. We even tried going on a cruise with all our family and friends that first year, but this was not a good thing for us either.

I know saying time heals all wounds is a cliché, but it's true. We needed time to process and deal with the depth of emotions we felt after that day and all the days that followed. While I will never forget the day he died, we have found it more effective to treat it as any other day.

We reached out to other people who had lost a child to suicide and they encouraged us to go to counseling. This was very good for me as it made me realize that Andrew dying by suicide did not mean that I failed him as a parent. He was ill, in a way that only he knew, and ultimately died because of mental illness.

In my final counseling session, I was told, "You're going to be fine." I asked, "How?" I couldn't imagine a day when I wasn't going to be in pain or when this loss didn't feel crippling. "You're not afraid to talk about it," the counselor told me. "You're not afraid to say he died by suicide, as opposed to committing suicide, which has a violent connotation. And you're not afraid to say your son was dealing with mental illness." That was the moment that I knew I could channel my grief and sadness into something positive.

Healing is ultimately about the survivors, not the lost. My grief was like a shoebox in a closet that I opened every day, then it became every other day, which turned into once a week, and now I open it only when I need to.

Call to Action

I remember the moment I decided to open up to other people about what I was going through. I was sitting in a bar one night and there was a guy beside me who started a conversation. I'd never met him before in my life, but I felt this urge to tell him the whole story. I opened up to a complete stranger about losing my son and it was an ah-ha moment for me. I realized that there is nothing to be embarrassed about. My son had mental illness. It's a disease and talking about it was good for me and for the person I was talking to.

I absorbed a lot of information about mental health the first year after Andrew passed. I also learned how suicidal thoughts and mental illness are so taboo that most people keep their suffering hidden, a secret they are embarrassed of and fear disclosing. The stigma of mental illness was so powerful that it keeps people from getting help. No other disease, especially one so treatable, is like that.

As I began to heal I wanted to do more, something more concrete that would fill those hours when my grief was too overwhelming. I wanted to find a way to be proactive and share my story with others. A friend introduced me to the Gracepoint Foundation, and I joined their board of directors in May of 2015. This opportunity has allowed me to connect to a special group of people, all with different connections to and experiences with to mental health and addiction, who wanted to get involved.

> Men make up over 75 percent of suicide victims in the United States, with one man killing himself every 20 minutes.
>
> Source: Psychology Today

Working with the Gracepoint Foundation over the last five years has allowed me to amplify my voice to spread mental health awareness. We started the Andrew Lutes Golf Outing in 2019 to help cultivate the endowment in Andrew's name and speak to the importance of mental health and suicide awareness. I am incredibly proud of the tremendous amount of financial support we have raised for the endowment, but more importantly the lives we have touched and families we have helped. The income generated from the endowment supports the critical services and programs for children at Gracepoint. If the support from our event or the endowment can save the life of even just ONE child, then somehow, someway, Andrew's death makes more sense.

I enjoy the advocacy work I do on my own as well, whether that's supporting those in need in my church community, spreading education and awareness on social media, speaking to groups, or reaching out to families who have lost a loved one to suicide. Young people today are under so many pressures and parents need to know the signs and when their kids may be in trouble. I want to provide value to anyone looking to learn more about mental health and help any parent seeking resources to support their child reaching out for help.

Being so open about my story has allowed me to connect with so many parents over concerns about their children. I'm always happy to share my story, take a call, or help direct them to the appropriate resources to navigate issues they are facing with their child. I feel I'm at a place in my healing where I can spread understanding and hope. I view it as a calling now.

Mental illness is a disease, not unlike cancer or heart disease; and, if left undiagnosed or untreated, it can be fatal. I want people to know that we must continue to educate ourselves about the signs of mental illness so we can be aware of them and prepared to deal with them. Building a community that is supportive of people who want to talk about mental illness removes the shame and encourages people to seek help without fear.

A little while after Andrew's death, I got a tattoo on my arm that says, "Everyone you meet is fighting a battle you know nothing about. Be kind. Always." It's a reminder to myself that sometimes, behind that beautiful smile and my son's big blue eyes, there was pain. Once we stop being afraid to talk about that pain, we can not only change lives, we can save them.

Paula Lutes

Corporate Lawyer, Fortune 500 Company

I know that any loss, particularly that of a child, changes you and makes you different than you were before. In the process, I'm not sure I even noticed that I had put my own feelings of grief and loss on the back burner.

My Story

The first thing I remember from that awful day, January 7, 2014, was the agonizing screams of my husband Bill. "Andrew's dead! Andrew's dead!"

In that next moment, I was spurred into action. I ran into the house and asked my parents to take our youngest son, Will, outside. I called 911 and remained unbelievably calm as I told the operator what happened. I was calm because someone had to be, and that someone was me.

A few minutes later, our house was a crime scene. The police taped off the area, began interviewing all of us, and investigated what had happened in the apartment over the garage where Andrew was staying. The detective and Bill went through all of Andrew's emails and his phone. The more we discovered, the more we saw a pattern emerge over the last few months; how Andrew avoided different things like exams and grad school. The story of what happened began to unfold.

I had called our priest to come over to console Bill and help figure out how we would break this horrific news to Andrew's mother and his older brother, Kyle, as well as the boys who lived with him at college. Throughout all of it, I kept telling myself that I couldn't fall apart, no matter what. There was so much to do, so many decisions to make, and we had a toddler who didn't understand what was going on.

At some point in the middle of the night, Bill and I turned to each other and realized, holy crap—we have to get up in the morning and celebrate a birthday. Andrew took his life the day before our son Will's third birthday. There was no way to explain to little Will that we couldn't celebrate his birthday; he'd been looking forward to it for weeks. That's how I knew Andrew was not well. He loved Will and, if he had thought about it, there's no way he would have taken his life the day before Will turned three.

So the next morning, we got up and had cupcakes for breakfast to celebrate Will's birthday. Unbeknownst to our young son, Bill and I were fighting the deepest and darkest pain imaginable. When people came over to our house to comfort us, Will thought they were there for his party. It was an unreal situation.

In the minutes, hours, and days after my stepson shot himself, I became sort of the air traffic controller who had to juggle multiple critical things at the same time and make sure no one else crashed. I just kept working to keep everything on track—from making arrangements to dealing with the paperwork—so I could allow Bill and Kyle the space to grieve.

I know that any loss, particularly that of a child, changes you and makes you different than you were before. In the process, I'm not sure I even noticed that I had put my own feelings of grief and loss on the back burner. I think it was the "for better or for worse" vow at its finest—I needed to be strong. How could I fall apart when Bill needed me?

Still, there was so much to go through in the days, weeks, and months after Andrew's suicide. The

90% of all people who die by suicide have a diagnosable psychiatric disorder at the time of their death.

Source: American Foundation for Suicide Prevention

more we dug into what was going on with him, the more we saw that he had felt this incredible pressure to live up to some impossible standard. It wasn't the people around him putting the pressure on him—it was Andrew himself. Andrew was a really special kid; he was a pleaser and never wanted to disappoint anyone. I think his reality had gotten so skewed that he thought he was somehow letting us all down and he couldn't see a way out.

I think of all the times he got down on the floor to play planes and cars with Will and what a sweet big brother he was. One of the greatest tragedies for me is that Will won't have the opportunity to get to know Andrew and, because he was so little, he won't even remember him.

When a child dies, it's truly the loss of a past, present and future. We lose all that was shared in the past, the immediate loss of their present life, and then the loss of what will never be in the future. I came into Andrew's life when he was a junior in high school and I'm certain he was skeptical and wary of me, having a new person enter his life. Slowly, we found our way and developed a mutual respect for each other.

Path to Wellness and Recovery

After Andrew died, I went through a long period of not really grieving. I'm a fixer, so I was in fix mode, keeping the wheels moving at the house with Will and our families. I was the one who had to keep making sure everyone was okay and that everything was on track. I think for stepparents, the grief experience becomes an uncertain and unstable journey as we try to balance the needs of our spouses, other family members, and our own feelings.

When a child loses a parent, we use the term "orphan" and when a husband or wife loses their spouse, we use the term "widow" or "widower". But there is no term to describe a parent who has lost a child and certainly nothing to describe a stepparent who experiences that loss. It was a friend in the mental health sector who described me as a "lost survivor" because, as a stepparent, I was almost always forgotten and the one whom some people thought didn't have a right to be so devastated about losing a child who was not biologically mine.

I would overhear people saying things like, "Oh, it was just her stepson," as if I didn't have a right to grieve losing him. I loved Andrew and I was devastated, too, when we lost him. Biological parent or not, my grief was real, my pain was real, and my sorrow continues.

Finding ways to cope with our grief and pain took on many forms. Bill and I did see a psychologist together a couple of times after Andrew died, but it took us some time to finally accept the loss. I tried a meditation app for a short while, but it did nothing for me. I found practicing self-care really helped and that exercise helped me feel better and stronger, both physically and mentally.

As a stepparent, after the death of a child you're an outsider and almost invisible to extended family, former spouses, other stepchildren, and even friends. My family and friends really rallied around me and helped me through my grief. I have always maintained a strong social network, a support system of close friends that I talk with almost every day. Having a strong friend group to talk to helped me express my grief in a healthy way. It was the human connection with my close friends that got me through the hardest days.

Will was a gift during this time. Having a young child gave me an outlet to pour all my energy into. When you have a three-year-old, you have to keep moving forward and it accelerated all of us getting back to reality and regular life.

One of my good friends lost her son to suicide a few months later and I was there, being the air traffic controller and keeping everything on track for her and, in a way, paying back all the friends who had been there for us.

Throughout all of this, I have found a place, and a voice, and a mission to try to protect any family and friends from enduring this pain alone in any way I could. Continuing to talk and help others is good for me. Being there for others helps me manage my own grief and I continue to move on from the deep sadness I used to feel. The deep sadness becomes less and less with time and painful moments happen less often.

As Bill began to transition from his feelings of profound loss, I began to feel better as well. Whenever I see a glimpse of joy appear on my husband's face again, I know I need to be even stronger because those happy moments are so precious. It's better now, our healing has come a long way, but we still miss Andrew so very much.

Call to Action

As a stepparent, you feel you are not worthy of the same grief as a biological parent. Even though I only knew Andrew for five years and not twenty-one, he was precious to me and I loved him dearly. For many stepparents, it can take real time to overcome the powerful feelings experienced after the loss of a child. But a willingness to share your experience—in a safe space with family or close friends—can, in time, lessen those feelings of sadness and isolation.

I want parents to please take the time to connect with your children—not over the phone or in a text—but face to face. Force them to be present even if they'd rather text than talk. Create a safe space that allows them to be vulnerable if they have fears or depression.

I continue to be a resource and speak to families in need. I put myself more front and center now concerning any discussion about mental health. I want everyone to encourage the people around them to be open about what they are going through and how they are feeling. The more we can connect and take away the stigma of mental illness, the more we can protect young lives so that no family has to feel this pain.

Our family host a golf event each year to raise money for endowment in Andrew's name, proceeds from the endowment go to support critical programs for children at Gracepoint. I proudly share my fondest memories of Andrew with our attendees and talk about the importance of mental health awareness, especially with our young people. Both Bill and I know that Andrew's story has the power to save lives, and though we will always miss our son, we are comforted that his story will continue to impact and help those in need.

When I think of Andrew, I think of him in the moments of happiness and joy, his beautiful blue eyes and contagious smile. Now I know that, behind that smile, he must have been suffering the deepest despair that none of us could understand. I choose, however, to remember his beautiful life and to make it my mission to encourage others to connect with their family and friends in meaningful ways.

There is a memorial for Andrew on the wall in the lobby of the Gracepoint Children's Crisis Center, next to his photo it reads: "Everyone you meet is fighting a battle you know nothing about. Be kind. Always."

> Every year in the United States, more than 45,000 people take their own lives. Every one of these deaths leaves an estimated six or more "suicide survivors" — people who've lost someone they care about deeply and are left with their grief and struggle to understand why it happened.
>
> Source: Harvard Health Publishing

Greg Baker

Chef and Restaurateur / Consultant, Chef Greg Baker Group

I'm honest and open with the fact that I'm still very much managing my depression and anxiety, and that manic phases still occur. I want people to feel free to say that they are not okay because there is no harm in that—it's human.

My Story

I was going through a really difficult time and had convinced myself there was no other way out—I was going to kill myself. I had a 357 handgun on the coffee table, loaded and ready; and then, out of nowhere, my dog Pandora comes over to where I was, curled up next to me, and put her head in my lap. It was an "I'm going to take everything bad away from you" type of gesture. She saved my life. I honor that moment and her memory with a tattoo of her paw print on my forearm.

I've considered suicide a couple of times in my life. The overwhelming stress of putting on a good face in tough times, having to take care of other people who depend on you, and being a leader with all the answers, can take a huge toll on you mentally. I struggled with negative thoughts all the time—*am I an imposter, am I going to screw up the next big event, should I be in the kitchen at all*—these questions were always at the back of my mind. It's an industry where you can feel a range of emotions from crushing loneliness to crippling anxiety, and all have the power to make you think that it might just be easier if you kill yourself to escape them.

I got initiated into the weird hours of restaurant life early, I was sixteen and working a middle-of-the-night shift at a 24-hour diner. I frequently worked from 5 p.m. to 3 a.m., or 11 p.m. to 7 a.m., even when I was in high school. When I got off work, my brain was still racing from the energy and fast pace of the shift. Until I could silence the activity in my head, I couldn't sleep. I'd have to get stoned and wait for the anxiety to go away, then I was calm enough to sleep.

I wandered around for a bit after high school. I tried college a couple of times and dropped out before I finally enrolled in culinary school. I started my career working in fine dining in Clearwater, but I ended up moving back to Portland, where I had lived before for a while. In the 80's, restaurant work wasn't exactly a glamorous profession, definitely not the way it is portrayed on television today. It was tough, the hours were long, and the environment in the kitchen was unforgiving.

When I left the restaurant late at night, even though I was physically exhausted, my brain was still in hyperdrive and it was impossible for me to rest. Those were the years when I really struggled with going home to an empty house, it was unbearably quiet. I didn't know what to do with those moments. My mind would fill with the rapid cycle of anxiety and depression, which just seemed to amplify the thoughts racing through my brain. My usual way of coping with it was to just drink myself to the point where my brain would shut up.

Drinking has been a part of my life almost since my first job, but I'd hated drinking when I first started working in restaurants. Part of the problem with the restaurant industry is that everything comes in waves. You'll have a little down time, then immediately transition to feeding a thousand people in just a few hours. The adrenaline keeps going, even after that last guest has left and you've scrubbed the kitchen. In this business, drinking is one of the few rewards you get at the end of the day. You have a great shift and you share a drink with your coworkers. You come to the end of the work week, you all toast together. Your new menu is a success, you pour some champagne for the entire staff. Consequentially, drinking and smoking become the primary tools used in this business to calm down and relax.

In 2017, approximately 2.3 million Americans between the ages of 12 and 17 and 2.4 million Americans between the ages of 18 and 25 started to drink alcohol.

Source: Addiction Center

One of the hardest things for me in the restaurant business is that we run on adrenaline at the times where most people are sleeping. When the rush is over and it's time to go home, our bodies are tired, but our minds are still running full-bore and we have no one to talk to about our day. You are then faced with what I call the "empty hour"—when you leave your restaurant late at night, your mind is still spinning and you can't yet rest. This was the loneliest time of day for me and when drinking became part of my daily routine.

In this industry, jobs don't offer benefit packages. We go without insurance—leaving people to self-fund any medical care—which usually means we go without care at all. It can become an expensive proposition to find out what's going on with your head and how to fix it. It took me thirty years to realize I had been self-medicating my undiagnosed bipolar disorder with alcohol. I don't necessarily call myself an alcoholic, but I am someone who is predisposed to drink too much when I'm not feeling well.

Path to Wellness and Recovery

I was discouraged the couple of times I decided to open up about my mental health to people that I thought would be supportive, but all I got back was, "You don't need that, you don't need to be on anti-depressants right now. You're fine," and even, "Wow, I always thought you were stronger than that." These types of judgmental and hurtful responses only made me feel more alone and my everyday struggle that much more challenging.

My wife and I owned a restaurant together, but a number of stressful things happened in a row (hurricane damage and a serial killer in our neighborhood) that hurt the business and put undue amounts of financial and mental stress on us both. When she stopped working evenings, I frequently got home later than normal and that empty hour was crushingly lonely and desperate for those couple of months. I resorted to drinking heavily on a daily basis and even tried to use social media to connect with humans who might still be awake because I was truly terrified to be alone with my thoughts. It had such a grip on me that it almost cost me my life.

Once I moved into management, I couldn't go out drinking with my coworkers or participate in staff after-work activities. That made me feel even lonelier. I would end up sitting alone at a bar just to have people around me while I drank. If you're craving social interaction, drinking in a bar becomes the socially acceptable answer. Around this time, I was in my late forties/early fifties and going out on the town or closing down a bar looked ridiculous. So, I would have a couple of drinks at the restaurant, go home and have a few more, all the while talking to myself about myself way too much. But after too many nights sitting on that bar stool and drinking by myself at home, I realized someone else was driving the bus in my brain.

After fighting to work through some tough situations, I reached out to other people in the industry about their routines to wind down and deal with that empty hour. I learned many of my colleagues were struggling as well and listened to how they addressed and managed their situations. I started opening up and talking about my mental health more, going to counseling, and doing rational emotive behavioral therapy (REBT). The goal of REBT is best described as challenging and questioning our irrational and dysfunctional beliefs and replacing them with more sensible and functional beliefs. I started to feel things were turning around for me.

I'm honest and open with the fact that I'm still very much managing my depression and anxiety, and manic phases still occur. At times, counseling has helped, but I prefer REBT. This therapy has given me more control over thoughts, so I can recognize when something is going wrong. My self-care and coping strategies have evolved over the years, as well. I find I really enjoy that time with my two dogs and walk one to three miles with them every day.

I could finally be honest with the people around me and that was like opening a door that I had been keeping shut for too long. I cut back on my drinking. I started exercising, meditating, and trying other methods to deal with and nurture my mental health. All of these things are pieces of a larger puzzle I used to cope. I realized, as with most things concerning mental health, there is no one-size-fits-all fix or treatment and I am always working to find what works best for me.

I don't know if people in the restaurant industry are predisposed to mental illness and addiction or not, but maybe the industry itself supports and nurtures it. There are a huge number of people I know in the industry who suffer from anxiety, depression, PTSD, and addiction. Several chefs have died by suicide and many more have been more open about their thoughts or attempts. Most of the general public knows about Anthony Bourdain's death by suicide, but there are many others whose stories don't make national news and that's why it's so important to talk about the toxic work culture, stress, and addiction associated with this line of work.

Call to Action

We sold the restaurant and I chose to retire. After thirty-five years, I've come to the realization that I can make a bigger impact in the world through writing and advocacy work than I ever could owning a restaurant and serving food. I feel that it's time to shift my focus to those areas. It's strange, but for the first time in my life I have Saturday nights off. My wife Michelle has been my support system, my life preserver, and I couldn't have made it this far without her.

I work in restaurant consulting now, while also doing some writing, and my life is a lot calmer. I now reach for a cup of tea rather than a shot of whiskey, and have found that trying to force myself to focus on a book for fifteen minutes is a mental exercise that shuts the thoughts down quicker than my old ways. I'm not afraid to try alternative therapies. In fact, I just finished a year micro-dosing mushrooms and I believe it has helped. Sometimes, rational thought and good life choices win; sometimes they don't. All I know is I'm now in a place where I have more good days than bad and that's an improvement, for sure.

I have become more open over the last ten years about my mental health and addiction. I'm definitely a work in progress. I started sharing my story because I don't want to see more people die because of their career choices or life circumstances. I've known too many good people who have died by suicide. I talk about my experiences with mental illness and addiction so people will realize they are not alone and can get help.

A good friend encouraged me to write about my story and experiences, and that's when I penned a column for *Food & Wine Magazine* called, "What to Do with the Empty Hour". I wrote the piece to open up about my mental health challenges, the stress of running a restaurant, and the issues harming the industry itself. Alcohol is ingrained in the restaurant culture (it

> 17% of food services workers have been diagnosed with a substance abuse disorder.
>
> Source: American Addiction Centers

almost encourages addiction) and there is a bigger tendency to drink than to talk about your problems.

I was fortunate to have the opportunity to be involved in a video piece from the *Wall Street Journal* called "Chefs Speak Out on Mental Health in the Restaurant Industry". The video uses personal testimonials to address the harsh work culture and stigma of mental illness in the restaurant industry. The video features prominent chefs like Cat Cora, Chris Cosentino, Charles Ford, Nirva Israel, and others who powerfully share their experiences and personal stories coping in an unforgiving and, at times, toxic industry.

People see mental illness as a character flaw and they can be so judgmental about it. Because of that, those who suffer are very hesitant to speak up and spend years in their own private hell before deciding to get help. It shouldn't have to be this way. We need to start filling those empty hours with positive conversations, understanding, and support.

I want people who suffer from mental illness to understand that this is something that is beyond their ability to control, but with help they can. Everyone needs to know that it's okay to not be okay. I know more than anyone how management is an everyday process. I'm very open about how I continue to manage with what I deal with inside my head and my efforts to keep it under control. It's not easy and there are no days off, but the results are worth it.

Those of us with lived experience and who have been through some dark times have an opportunity to pave the way for change through our shared stories. I like the saying, "What has always been does not have to always be." I want people to feel free to say that they are not okay because there is no harm in that—it's human. The more stories shared about mental health, the more public discussion, the less stigma will be attached to it. The result will be more people getting the help they need.

Johnny Crowder

Founder & CEO, Cope Notes / Professional Musician

*Anyone and everyone can have mental illness,
and the more we talk about it, the more we realize
that we are all going through this together.*

My Story

Like all too many others, I grew up in a home surrounded by drugs and alcohol, where I endured a wide variety of abuse. At a very young age, I learned that my life was of little value, and that a majority of my experiences would undoubtedly end with some kind of pain. I even tried to take my own life because, for years, I saw death as the only viable solution to my suffering.

I was hallucinating, counting my steps, obsessing over germs, and contemplating suicide on a minute-to-minute basis. As you can imagine, this made connecting with other people a little challenging. I had a small, tight-knit friend group, but there were times when I would recoil from them, and others when I needed company so desperately that I wouldn't leave a friend's house unless by force. Deep down, I knew that going home meant returning to an unsafe environment to be alone with my thoughts. Again.

After a particularly extreme outburst at the age of fifteen, my mother gave me a choice: Start treatment the easy way or the hard way. "Do you want me to drive you there, or would you rather have the police take you?" she asked.

The doctor gave me a laundry list of diagnoses. It was like the whole alphabet. I stared at the floor while he gave me the "we can help" speech, and tried to make sense of what he was saying. Schizophrenia? OCD? PTSD? Bipolar? Are you serious? Are you going put me in a straitjacket or something? That's not me, is it?

I felt doomed and helpless. So helpless that all I could do was have healthy people with diplomas on their walls give me medicine until I was too bloated to roll out of bed. There was a part of me that wanted to know more, call it morbid curiosity or sheer desperation, but I wanted to learn more about what I was experiencing. So when I went away to college I studied psychology.

From those studies, I learned, as it turns out, nothing was "wrong" with me at all and that mental illness was not as simple as we have made it out to be after generations of stereotyping it. With each lecture, I slowly unlearned the stereotypes I had picked up from books, movies, and TV shows growing up; the very same ones that struck fear in me the moment I was diagnosed.

Path to Wellness and Recovery

My childhood diagnoses still persist to this day, but the symptoms manifest to varying degrees of severity. While I'm no longer medicated, I did recently begin seeing a therapist again in light of COVID-19 and all of the mental and emotional stressors that came with it.

I feel like a brand new person these days, but it hasn't been an easy road. It took years of deep critical thinking, treatment, studying, relationship building, hard work, and faith for me to begin taking responsibility for my mental health on a regular basis. I am very fortunate to be alive today, and I refuse to take that for granted. Keeping my brain healthy is just my way of preserving this new lease on life that I've been gifted.

Every day, I discover a new way to practice self-care that contradicts my mental image of what self-care should look like. Some days, self-care means scrolling through social media to find videos of my favorite supercars, while other days it means not touching social media at all. I've tried all sorts of things, from rearranging my living room furniture to watching documentaries about sneakers. I think a lot of us get too wrapped up in making sure that our techniques look like self-care rather than focusing on whether or not they actually feel like it.

Yes, I see a therapist, I read books about personal development and positive psychology, I take deep breaths, I exercise regularly and pray every day…there's a lot of validity to these things. But some nights, I pour myself a bowl of cereal for dessert because allowing

> About 7 or 8 out of every 100 people (or 7-8% of the population) will have PTSD at some point in their lives.
>
> Source: U.S. Department of Veterans Affairs

myself to enjoy comfort food is another step forward in my eating disorder recovery.

One thing that helped me shed my fear of judgment and pursue advocacy was, oddly enough, improv comedy. Teaching and performing helped me get out of my own head and become more comfortable with being vulnerable in front of other people. On an improv stage, you have to be unafraid to look, act, and sound like a total weirdo. No one can be "normal" when they're playing some ridiculous character that the audience made up on the spot.

Music was just as helpful, if not more. When I first started performing, I couldn't even look out into the crowd or make eye contact with my band members. Over time, I had to break out of my shell or risk losing my favorite creative outlet. It was a real "adapt or perish" situation, but the strength and freedom that music has afforded me was well worth fighting for.

As I started opening up about my mental health more and more in my music, fans began lining up after the show just to share their experiences and tell me how they can relate. I expected people to poke fun at me for being weak, for being vulnerable. Instead, I was met with compassion, empathy, and a community the likes of which I never thought I'd find in dark, dingy bars and venues all across the country.

At the end of the day, we need to remember that self-care means giving ourselves enough grace to nurture all of the corners of our personality, not just the ones we publicly associate with mental and emotional health.

Call to Action

My advice to anyone—start where you are. I know that most people wouldn't consider death metal to be the most conventional vehicle for advocacy. But as my most trusted and comfortable outlet for creativity and self-expression, it was the perfect starting place for me.

Cultural norms have taught us how to think about mental health, but it's time to take the conversation back into our own hands. For two decades, I was convinced that other people wouldn't be interested in my story. I didn't think that mine was pretty enough. I couldn't wrap it up in a bow like celebrities do during talk-show appearances. Mine was downright ugly.

But the more I opened up, the more I wanted to find a way to expand the conversation around mental health, even if it meant putting myself out there and taking big risks.

I created a mental health platform called Cope Notes back in 2018, and we've reached thousands upon thousands of people in just a few short years with our podcast, presentations, and daily text messages. All I wanted to do was invent a way to interrupt negative thought patterns and teach people to improve their mental health. Now, keep in mind: I'm no tech maven. I'm a regular person, just like you, who decided that they couldn't sit on the sidelines any longer.

Mental health is universal. Cope Notes has users in almost 100 countries, which blows my mind to this day. When you're dealing with your own issues, it's easy to forget that there are millions of people out there who can relate. As we continue to spark these conversations, we will come to realize that we're all going through this together.

> National prevalence data indicate that nearly 40 million people in the United States (18%) experience an anxiety disorder in any given year.
>
> Source: Anxiety and Depression Association of America

When I started the Cope Notes podcast, I thought my primary audience would be young people, but it turns out our listeners are mature adults and working professionals. Our audience is comprised of a wide variety of ethnicities, ages, gender identities, and people from many countries. These conversations are slowly starting to change the stigma around mental health and I think part of it is because we are all connected to each other's stories.

I set out to change the health conversation to equally include both its mental and physical aspects. Wellness is not just about physical health—it's about mental health, too. For years, I'd wanted to do a TEDx talk but had no idea how people got chosen to present. A lot of us disqualify ourselves from opportunities like that. After all, I'm not a doctor; I'm just a twenty-seven-year-old guy who has a lot of tattoos. When I was accepted to be a speaker at TED˟Eustis, I was overwhelmed. *"How to Grow as a Person and Why it Sucks"* aired in February of 2020 and I've been very pleasantly surprised at the amount of people who have seen it, shared it, or mentioned it to me.

Whatever you love, whatever you're passionate about, I guarantee you there's a way to leverage it for the good of the people around you. For me, it's been music, comedy, art, writing, speaking… the list goes on. At first, I was nervous to reveal too much of myself, to my surprise, weaving my personality and story into our music and performances has only enriched the experience for me and our listeners by tenfold.

You might not think that a connection can be drawn between your story and your passion, but I'm living proof that anything is possible if you give enough of a crap about it. No matter what you feel called to do, there is a way to inject your personality and truth into it. And if you do that, carefully and with the right intentions, a whole lot of people can stand to benefit from your authenticity…including you.

A Thank You Story

I want to express my gratitude to all of our contributors for agreeing to share their stories as part of our effort to address and end the stigma surrounding mental illness and addiction. These stories are meant to inspire anyone who has suffered grief and loss, struggled to seek help, in recovery, or looking for a way to get involved to help others. Thank you again for supporting mental health and addiction awareness. This is a book I know you will be proud of—one that will positively impact the lives of many for years to come.

As a special thank you to the individuals who gave so much of themselves to share their story, I would like to dedicate to them a poem by Alberto Rios, written in 1952.

When Giving Is All We Have

One river gives
Its journey to the next.

We give because someone gave to us.
We give because nobody gave to us.

We give because giving has changed us.
We give because giving could have changed us.

We have been better for it,
We have been wounded by it—

Giving has many faces: It is loud and quiet,
Big, though small, diamond in wood-nails.

Its story is old, the plot worn and the pages too,
But we read this book, anyway, over and again:

Giving is, first and every time, hand to hand,
Mine to yours, yours to mine.

You gave me blue and I gave you yellow.
Together we are simple green. You gave me

What you did not have, and I gave you
What I had to give—together, we made

Something greater from the difference.

A Call to Action for Family and Friends

A Story YOU Need to Hear

One of the scariest things for anyone feeling depressed, overwhelming sadness, or having suicidal thoughts—is to tell another person they are feeling that way. The fear of being judged harshly, criticized, or even ridiculed is real for most people. What can be even worse is receiving that reaction from those we care about the most: our family and friends. This is one of the main reasons people wait so long to disclose their suffering.

It's worth repeating what I mentioned earlier in the introduction: Everyday people—working professionals, retired seniors, and students alike—fear losing, if they disclose, the three things that matter the most to them in their life: their family, their friends, and their jobs. This is why family and friends can have the most impact in abating this fear, but some real work needs to be done before that can happen.

> ## The average delay between symptom onset and treatment is eleven years.
>
> Source: National Alliance on Mental Illness

The front line of support for many of us when something goes wrong is our family and friends. We turn to this group when we get a cancer diagnosis, experience the loss of a loved one, or are rushed to the emergency room. But where mental illness is concerned–that is where our comfort level ends. For many, the period of time between discovering an issue and getting help is heartbreaking, unhealthy, and sometimes dangerous. Jobs are lost, relationships end, drugs and alcohol are prevalent, and for many the probability of self-harm is real.

We often put family and close friends on a pedestal and never want to see each other as weak or hurting. Because of this, so often our first reaction to an issue is not the best. Family and friends sometimes default to misconceptions and myths about mental illness, which leads to a breakdown in not only communication, but in many cases the relationship itself. In addition to the common six myths mentioned about mental illness earlier in the book, with those closest to us we have the tendency to shift to even more negative and hurtful statements, such as saying those who disclose just want attention or are using their illness to manipulate those around them.

Moving from a comfort level that is unsure how to support someone with mental illness to one that is relaxed and composed takes practice and consistency over time. Family and friends have to understand a few important elements about how to support someone struggling:

- Be patient with the one suffering. People grieve and feel depressed on their own timeline. No amount of support or cheering up will change that.

- Do not attempt to diagnose. Remember you are there to be a friend and supporter, not a doctor. It's always good to read up on mental illness to be better informed and understand potential triggers and behaviors.

- Remind the person how much they mean to you. Being with someone suffering, present and available, usually means more to them than you know. But we have to also remember to give them space if they ask.

- Help to offer with daily task items, like cooking, cleaning, or going to the store if they are struggling or unmotivated to get them done.

- When looking after someone with a mental illness, remember to look after your own mental health as well. No one can pour from an empty cup.

Being able to have a conversation about mental illness is a great way to grow within your comfort level to support a loved one who is struggling. A good way to begin this conversation is to start by saying, "How can I help," and then listening without judgment. As a loved one, the ability to listen is so important. We have to listen with intention to understand their situation, not to fix it. Responding is just as important. It's best to respond in a way that validates their feelings and empathizes with their situation. Never downplay their situation or jump in with solutions you feel will solve their problem. Helping someone struggling with their mental health has a lot to do with effective communication designed to support the one suffering, not antagonize them.

Friends and family have powerful roles to play in supporting those in need of support for a mental health or addiction problem. The problem is not the same for everyone, although mental health issues do not discriminate—people do—and these reactions to a disclosure for help can cause a lot of harm. As the support system for our loved ones we have to educate ourselves on more than just mental health, we have to better understand the cultural and societal barriers keeping people from getting help or having access to it.

Path to Wellness and Recovery

Friends and family can be great advocates and caregivers, but there still needs to be a more proactive approach when it concerns the issue of suicide. According to the National Institute of Mental Health (NIMH), suicide is the tenth leading cause of death overall in the United States. With all the overwhelming data around—suicidal ideation, self-harm, suicide attempts, and number of suicides each year—an alarm should be sounding somewhere and this issue addressed more on a national stage, yet little is said in the media. Awareness and education are nonexistent to both our teachers and our students, and corporate employee wellness plans rarely address it, leaving the need for friends and family support and advocacy higher than ever.

According to the Center for Disease Control and Prevention (CDC), the suicide rate from 1999 through 2017 in the U.S. increased 33%.

We have to recognize that not every demographic group has the same options or cultural awareness concerning mental health services. There have been increased rates of suicide in some marginalized communities which need to be addressed. Black, Indigenous, and people of color (BIPOC) communities and Lesbian, Gay, Bisexual, Transgender, Queer/Questioning (LGBTQ) people are often misunderstood, overlooked, and underrepresented in the health care system. These groups have disproportionate access to mental health services because of issues of stigma, cultural and socioeconomic barriers, and an overall lack of awareness about mental health.

African Americans have been and continue to be negatively affected by prejudice and discrimination in the health care system. Inadequate treatment and lack of cultural competence by health professionals cause distrust and prevent many from seeking treatment or trusting what is available. According to research from NAMI, BIPOC communities are suffering from mental health issues at a higher rate compared to the U.S. average.

- African Americans are 20% more likely to experience mental health issues than the rest of the population.

- Native Americans between the ages of 18 and 24 have the highest suicide rates of any ethnic group, and 40% of the individuals who die by suicide are between 15 and 24 years old.

- Only 2.3% of black or Hispanic young people see a professional for mental health issues every year compared to 5.7% of white children.

Mental health conditions do not discriminate based on gender identity or sexual orientation, however, they both can make access to mental health services more problematic and difficult. LGBTQ individuals often suffer from poor mental health outcomes due to difficulty finding quality support services, discrimination, and homophobia. LGBTQ youth and young adults are disproportionately harassed, bullied, and victims of hate crimes compared to other groups. Because of this, according to NAMI, LGBTQ youth experience higher risk of mental health and addiction related issues:

- Are nearly 2X as likely as heterosexual adults to experience a substance use disorder.

- Are almost 5X as likely to attempt suicide compared to their heterosexual peers.

- Lesbian, gay, and bisexual youth are 4X more likely to attempt suicide than straight youth.

- 40% of transgender adults have attempted suicide in their lifetime, compared to less than 5% of the general U.S. population.
- Have a 120% higher risk of experiencing homelessness.

LGBTQ individuals are two times more likely than others to experience a mental health condition such as major depression or generalized anxiety disorder. Though more therapists and counselors today have positive attitudes toward the LGBTQ community, many still face unequal care due to a lack of training and understanding. Additionally, some in the LGBTQ community may face harassment or a lack of cultural competency from potential providers. Because of the potential discrimination or provider bias, these experiences have kept those who receive treatment fearful of disclosing their sexual orientation or gender identity.

Understanding cultural and societal barriers to services and support is the first step in addressing these issues directly. Providers, caregivers and loved ones have a long way to go to become more culturally competent, but as allies to these groups we can do a lot to change these prejudices and help remove the stigma attached to them. There is no better group to show this support to them than family and friends. We have the power to speak out against discriminatory language and actions—to create supportive and inclusive environments at school, work and home. Confronting these barriers is within our power and can lead to better mental health outcomes and support recovery.

Call to Action

Most of us are hard-wired to want to help anyone we care about who is hurting or says they need help. With mental illness we just have to approach things a little differently, and understand how powerful actions like listening, encouragement, and even helping navigate resources can be for someone in need. Taking the time to learn about mental health and addiction is so important, the more we know and understand, the more we can empathize with our loved ones.

Mental health is complicated and solutions, like medication and therapy, will not fix anything overnight. We have to understand even the little things like visiting someone, starting a conversation, or celebrating small steps in their recovery are all things we can do to be supportive in someone's mental health journey.

As friends and family, we have to make suggesting going to see a therapist or counselor when someone says they are feeling overwhelmed, experiencing grief, or having suicidal thoughts as normal as going to the doctor when someone says they are sick or hurt. We have to encourage and even sometimes start the conversation. We have to understand and help others to understand that there is nothing wrong with experiencing a mental health problem and that it is okay to express how you are feeling. Talking about mental health shows strength and courage, and hiding mental health problems can make things worse.

Taking on the challenges linked to mental health whether it is availability to services for all, affordable health care coverage, or the stigma associated with it, requires all of us. Together we have to push back on the idea that someone needs to hit rock bottom in order to receive support for their mental health. I challenge everyone who has a loved one who experiences a mental health issue in the future to pause from saying things like, "you'll get over it" or "don't be so sad," and just say "I believe you." These three words have the power to change a conversation and even save a life.

It can be hard to see a friend or family member in a different light after they have disclosed a mental illness or addiction. Please try to understand the hopelessness, isolation, loneliness, and darkness they are going through. It can be hard to be a friend to someone suffering, but it also can be the kindest and most supportive thing you ever do. If you know someone who is suffering from a mental illness—my call to action to you—as a member of their family and support system is to remember—if you can be anything, please be patient and kind.

Special shout out to all the allies, family members, and close friends who support a loved one in suffering or in recovery. Your love, patience, and unwavering support are seldom recognized. You've been helping those in need win battles and transform their lives in an effort to manage their mental illness or recover from addiction. Keep going, keep advocating, keep educating others—you are helping move this conversation in the right direction. More importantly—your actions save lives.

A Call to Action for Men

A Story About Men's Mental Health

The need to end stigma and make mental health a priority for men has never been greater. Today, men are dying by suicide at an alarming rate. Suicide has become a silent killer of men that is rarely discussed publicly, even though the research tells us that men are nearly four times more likely to die by suicide than women. According to the American Foundation for Suicide Prevention, men account for almost 70% of all suicides.

Men who are vocal about their mental health issues are usually dismissed by their peers and family as weak, flawed, or even broken. It is this label and mark of disgrace that defines what makes up the stigma associated with mental illness. Stigma is particularly dangerous for men because they are less likely to seek help and more likely than women to turn to dangerous or unhealthy behaviors, such as drugs or alcohol, as a means of coping with their mental health challenges.

Approximately 15.1% of adult American men were diagnosed with some type of mental illness in 2017.

Source: National Institute of Mental Health

The two words that have prevented more men from seeking the help they really need are "man up". Research tells us that, from the time they are children until adulthood, men receive messages that discourage them from ever letting anyone know how they feel. Men have had an overall misconception about mental health that has led to the powerful stigma associated with it, the outcome of which has been attributed to long-term suffering, destructive behavior, and even death. Because of this, it is difficult for men to talk to anyone or take charge of their own mental health.

Three of the biggest myths that get between men and their mental health include:

1. "Depression isn't real": Depression is a real medical condition that can affect your body, thoughts, emotions, and behaviors. It's different from normal sadness in that it consumes your everyday life and interferes with your ability to work, eat, sleep, and have fun. When depressed, the feelings of being helpless, hopeless, and worthless can be intense.

2. "Feeling depressed means you are weak": Suffering from depression has nothing to do with your personal strength. It is a serious health condition that millions of men struggle with each year and it can happen to anyone. Men need to know that mental illness is a disease, not unlike heart disease or cancer; and, if left undiagnosed or untreated, it can be fatal.

3. "Real men don't ask for help": Ignoring depression doesn't make it go away. Consulting a professional who has more knowledge about depression and treatment options is the smartest thing someone suffering can do. Talking to a therapist is a proven treatment for depression.

Men struggle with the idea of being vulnerable and sharing their emotions because certain ideas about masculinity are drilled into them at an early age. Toxic masculinity is very real. Researchers have defined it, in part, as a set of behaviors and beliefs that include the following: Suppressing emotions or masking distress, maintaining an appearance of hardness, and violence as an indicator of power. Toxic masculinity is what can come from teaching boys and young men that they shouldn't openly express their emotions or feelings.

Growing up, those labeled as "sensitive boys" are often teased and ridiculed for what are natural and healthy expressions of emotion. This makes it even harder for those kids to talk about negative thoughts when they reach adulthood. This often leaves most men only reaching out for help when they feel they've hit "rock bottom" and others don't seek help at all.

No other illness is more impacted by stigma than mental illness. We rush to sign a cast on a broken leg but steer clear of anyone who tells us they feel depressed. The fear of disclosing a mental health issue is real because it brings with it a fear of being labeled by the illness. Unfortunately, the reaction most men receive when speaking to close friends and family about a mental illness is usually unforgiving and unsympathetic, and it can be very damaging. This can keep men from seeking help for years, if at all.

Path to Wellness and Recovery

Although men and women both suffer from mental illness, men are a lot less likely to reach out for help and often struggle in silence for years. Battling depression and suicidal thoughts is difficult and there is no question that it can be hard to talk about. Ultimately, for men it's the shame and fear they feel that prevents them from seeking any help or treatment.

A range of factors and experiences can contribute to the development of mental health challenges in men. These can include:

- Experiencing childhood abuse and family issues.
- Loss of work: Unemployment and retirement are associated with an increased risk of depression in men.
- Financial issues: Money pressures are a top cause of stress for many people and could play a role in the development of certain mental health disorders.
- Trauma: This could include extreme emotional events such as being sexually abused, experience in combat, witnessing a violent event, or being in high-stress situations on a regular basis.
- Separation and divorce: Depression is more prevalent and more severe among divorced men.

Today, educating men about mental health has never been more important. Every man needs to understand the symptoms of depression and how they can present themselves. The trademark symptoms of depression can include fatigue or decreased energy, difficulty concentrating or making decisions, insomnia, changes in weight from decreased or increased appetite, feelings of worthlessness or guilt, and a loss of interest in activities. While men can and do suffer from all of these, they can also experience symptoms that are more difficult to recognize and diagnose as depression. These can include increased irritability, working too much, increased substance abuse through drugs or alcohol, and increased risk taking. Because these symptoms are associated with normal masculine traits and can be seen as positive characteristics, men who are struggling in silence are often overlooked.

Seeking treatment is one of the most important and effective ways people with mental illness can improve the quality of their lives. For men it takes consistency of message, encouragement, and a little patience for this to happen. Treatment can provide a number of important benefits, such as:

90% of those who died by suicide had a diagnosable mental health condition at the time of their death.

Source: American Foundation for Suicide Prevention

- Helping you understand your condition.
- Reducing symptoms and improving your quality of life.
- Helping improve your relationships with family and friends.
- Reducing or eliminating negative or destructive behaviors.
- Peer support and group counseling can be particularly helpful and can help destigmatize mental illness.

What will it take to reduce the stigma associated with mental illness so that men will seek help instead of self-harming? It starts with men acknowledging their depression, understanding that they are more than their diagnoses, and then making the important changes in their lives to manage the illness. It takes men willing to share their stories of lived experience and recovery in order to help change the discussion from one of shame to one that's supportive. Finally, I believe men need to understand that addressing mental illness is not showing weakness. It takes courage and strength and, most of all, a lot of hard work—and these are all qualities of strong people.

Call to Action

Mental health issues are a lot more common than most people think and it's going to take more men willing to speak up to end stigma and support a culture of acceptance around getting help. This is so important because society isolates too many men by the norms they are supposed to adhere to. Men have emotions and feelings, just like everyone else; they do not always have to believe they need to be the tough ones in the room. We have to start normalizing things for men, like asking for help, going to therapy, expressing feelings, showing emotion, and seeking help for mental health concerns.

The stigma and shame associated with men's mental health keeps too many from getting the help they need. Suffering in silence is not a safe option for men anymore. Men don't always show the signs we often associate with depression, like sadness and hopelessness, but if you think someone you love is suffering—offer your support, listen, and be patient. Encourage him to talk to his doctor, a mental health professional, or help him find available behavioral health services.

As a society, we have to remember that men can and do suffer traumatic experiences that may greatly impact their mental health. That men have unresolved trauma and experience suicidal thoughts. That men do suffer from abuse and can be bullied. Men feel anxiety and depression. We have to talk more about these traumas, break down the stigma attached to them, and encourage men to get help.

For men, it starts with acknowledging they need help. There are two crucial steps—accepting that they need to make essential changes to manage their mental health or recovery and then doing that every day. This takes an incredible amount of discipline, consistency, courage, and strength. There will be good days and bad days, but know that it can be done. You've got this!

Men need to be a big part of today's movement to address mental health. They need to support one another when they share their story and encourage more men to do the same. We all have the responsibility to call out and shout down those voices who shame or ridicule men for showing emotion and sharing their feelings. We need to do our best to create and protect those safe spaces needed for men who have yet to disclose. More importantly, men need to understand the importance of mental health because, for them, it could be a matter of life and death.

A Call to Action for the Business Sector

A Corporate Sector Story

Understanding how mental health impacts organizations through reduced productivity, absenteeism, low employee engagement, and increased employee attrition are just a few of the reasons corporate leaders need to address the issue of mental health in the workplace. We have learned from research over the years that an employee's mental health greatly affects both their work performance and the company's financial bottom line. According to the Centers for Disease Control and Prevention (CDC), depression affects more than 17 million Americans and results in 200 million lost workdays in the U.S. annually.

Individuals who don't seek treatment can have a negative impact on their company because of the decline in their workplace performance and productivity. Studies continue to show that there are more workdays lost and more work injuries caused by mental illness than any other chronic health condition, including arthritis, diabetes, heart disease, and back pain. The CDC reports that about 80% of adults with depression reported at least some difficulty with work, home, or at social activities because of their depression symptoms, and 60% of employees have never spoken to anyone at work about their mental health.

Depression costs the U.S. economy $210.5 billion per year in absenteeism, decreased productivity, and medical costs.

Source: The Center for Workplace Mental Health

It's critical that companies recognize that mental health is just as important as physical health. Companies who invest and prioritize mental health, wellness, and self-care can help create a healthier work culture for their employees. These investments can show significant improvement in employee retention and engagement while cultivating the type of work environment that will attract top talent. Where so many companies fall short is how to act and where to start, but both research and employees are saying the time is now.

According to the CDC, the workplace is an optimal setting to create a culture of health because of the following:

- Communication structures are already in place.

- Programs and policies come from one central team.

- Social support networks are available.

- Employers can offer incentives to reinforce healthy behaviors.

- Employers can use data to track progress and measure the effects.

A 2019 Harvard study surveyed 1,500 people from each generational group and it showed that half of the Millennials and 75% of the Gen Zers said they had left jobs in the past for mental health reasons. With Millennials or Gen Z making up 75% of the current total workforce in the U.S., this study confirms a shift in focusing on mental health awareness. These two generational groups are also now prioritizing workplace culture, mental health and wellness programs, and benefits when choosing a company to work for.

It's important for business leaders to not only take this issue seriously—but to take action. However, many executives and managers still believe an employee's mental health is none of their concern or responsibility. As mental health becomes more of a focus in corporate culture, studies continue to hone in on the impact mental illness has on the business sector and why companies should be concerned.

The American Heart Association CEO Roundtable commissioned a report in 2020 to underscore the business imperative employers have for providing comprehensive, science-based support for employee mental health. A national poll of U.S. employees, conducted by Harris Poll for the CEO Roundtable, found a prevalence of mental health disorders:

- Roughly three in four employees (76%) indicate they have struggled with at least one issue that affected their mental health.

- About two in five employees (42%) answered yes when asked if they have ever been diagnosed with a mental health disorder.

- Although many were willing to divulge their disorder in this confidential survey, 63% of those diagnosed with a disorder say they have not disclosed it to their employer.

The American Heart Association CEO Roundtable Harris Poll also asked about perceptions of the employer's role around mental health:

- Nearly nine in ten survey respondents agree that employers have a responsibility to support mental health. Although more than eight in ten employees say their employers provide at least one mental health offering, they also say those employers can do more.

- 42% of employees would like their employers to provide more information about mental health benefits, accommodations, and resources.

- 40% want their employers to train managers and supervisors to identify emotional distress among workers.

For the last couple of years, corporations and the business community have debated how to address their employees' growing need and desire for more support. While tackling mental health can be challenging, organizations and executive leaders are in a powerful position to help change attitudes and offer a vital support system. Mental health is quickly becoming the next frontier of human resource department programing and employees want their company cultures to reflect this desire for change.

The Path to Employee Wellness and Support

Mental health challenges are a growing concern for employers all over the world. There are a lot of ways managers and leaders can connect with their teams to help build a mental health-friendly atmosphere and culture at work. The fear most have is not understanding mental health issues enough to feel confident in reaching out to someone suffering and discuss it. Leaders today have the responsibility to look after their people and that requires two very important elements— continuing education and the willingness to leave their comfort zones.

Now, more than ever, it's essential to educate managers and employees alike about mental health resources and the importance of nurturing an environment of openness at work in regards to mental health. Shifting a culture to focus more on mental health so employees feel safe disclosing an issue doesn't happen overnight. Employees know when these types of efforts are not genuine or authentic and, unfortunately, all too often this is where many fall flat. To cultivate a culture of empathy, psychological safety, and wellness, requires consistency and effort, with a strong focus on three major themes— environment, encouragement, and promotion.

Environment: Includes the surroundings and conditions in which your employees operate and function on a daily basis. Start by including behavioral health in your company's overall wellness plan and consider investing in mental health education. Mental Health First Aid training is a great place to start, and managers and leaders can be certified for two years after one eight-hour training session. This program provides training in mental health literacy, risk factors, and warning signs for mental health and addiction as well as strategies for how to provide help to someone in a crisis situation.

Encouragement: The action of giving someone support, confidence, or approval is imperative. New managers struggle with encouragement—it takes training and practice—and for some that is out of their comfort zone. Trainings on conflict resolution, stress management, and Mental Health First Aid can support and cultivate the skills needed to effectively approach employees and coworkers. It's essential to support any employee's effort to seek treatment for a mental health issue. Making an effort to start a dialogue is not only the best way to support and encourage employees, but to win them over as well.

Promotion: The consistent and ongoing work put in after the events and workshops to keep employees involved in supporting and looking out for each other. To effectively support a culture that values employee mental health and wellness, leadership must not only champion these efforts, but actively participate as well.

Employees want their managers to show empathy and concern. These actions build trust and loyalty with their teams. Encourage employees to schedule time off, especially after time-consuming projects, so they don't become overworked. If you notice someone struggling, engage them in conversation right away so they know you are looking after them and can address whatever the issue may be, sooner rather than later. One of the best strategies to support mental health is regularly scheduled one-on-one meetings with the members of your team—not just to focus on work, but to see how they are doing.

The time is now to support employee mental health and promote wellness initiatives. The corporate sector has an opportunity to take advantage of a climate for change to meet the demands of today's workforce. Promoting mental health and self-care can have a positive impact on a company in many ways, including addressing issues concerning employee retention and engagement, staff morale, and recruiting new talent. But the number one reason to promote mental health is to take care of your employees.

Employees who feel safe and cared for at work—and feel the company is looking out for their best interests—are more productive... more loyal...and more engaged!

A Call to Action

Normalizing conversations about mental health is the best way to reduce the stigma within the workplace. The goal for managers should be to promote the acceptance and inclusion of those dealing with mental health related issues by improving support systems for this population, spreading awareness whenever possible, and creating safe environments for discussion and education to take place.

By providing educational opportunities and enhancing awareness of mental illness and addiction through discussion, organizations are reducing the stigma which keeps employees silent in their suffering. Here are four strategies that any size company can incorporate, with little to no financial investment, in order to help cultivate a culture of empathy and support around mental health.

1. Make sure employees know it's safe for them to discuss and address mental health related issues by doing the following:

   - Provide safe environments, both in person and online, to discuss and educate the staff on mental health related topics, psychological safety, and wellness.

   - Create and include a written mental health non-discrimination statement in the employee handbook.

   - Allow employees more flexibility in their work schedule for any who are suffering from grief and loss or a diagnosed mental illness. These flexibility options can include working nontraditional hours, compressed work weeks, and telecommuting.

2. Share stories across all levels of personal experience, lived experience (living with a diagnosed mental illness), and recovery.

   - This precedent should be set by executives, managers, and other company leaders.

   - When leaders are vulnerable and share their experiences, or the experiences of those closest to them, it helps create transparency and acceptance in the workplace.

   - Sharing stories makes it easier for employees to ask for help when they need it; these stories can help take the fear out of their own disclosure.

3. Educate employees and managers about mental illness.

   - Promote mental health through in-service trainings, panel discussions, and workshops on mental health awareness and how to recognize signs of stress and poor mental health.

   - Train managers and supervisors to be aware of the signs of mental health issues and how to respond to them appropriately.

- Strive for a supportive work culture and a stigma-free workplace by regularly addressing mental health, as well as utilizing national recognition days and months on the calendar.

4. Make wellness a priority.
    - Establish and promote an Employee Assistance Program (EAP).
    - Encourage work/life balance and promote exercise, healthy eating, and participation in leisure activities to improve mental health.
    - Wellness programs can bring employees together and foster a friendly competitiveness in the office.

Managers and executive teams have the capability to support their employees with dignity and empathy. By providing safe environments to discuss, educate, and promote mental health and wellness, managers can cultivate the kind of work culture that can have a positive impact on a number of important organizational issues, including employee retention and engagement, staff morale, and the recruitment of top talent.

According to a study published in 2016 by *The Lancet Psychiatry*, for every $1 spent on mental health treatment such as counseling and medication, governments could receive a $4 return on their investment.

There is a clear business case to be made for the corporate sector to promote and invest in mental health awareness and self-care with their employees. Many Fortune 500 companies have started to implement efforts to attract top talent and improve the overall employee experience.

By shining a light on the alarming economic cost of mental illness, research groups have encouraged those in the corporate sector to be more proactive and implement policies that can better support their employees overall mental health and wellbeing.

The Power of Collective Voice

Thank you…for finding time in your busy life to become a part of a shared story. For creating a safe space to hear and talk about a powerful, and at times difficult, subject matter. For being willing to challenge preconceived ideas and beliefs. For purchasing this book to support mental health awareness and services. For hopefully sharing this book with another when you are finished. Thank you.

Everyone should have the ability and opportunity to share their voice. Like many, I struggled for years to express the heartbreak I felt over how addiction and mental illness had impacted my family and close friends. But in the wake of that pain has come a purpose and a willingness to be vocal, share my story, and continue to encourage others to do the same. Silence is not an option. Everyone deserves to have their voice heard.

You can't get over mental illness by ignoring it. You recover from it by cultivating a life where it becomes easier to manage; that's where you ultimately find a path to wellness. Once you are on that path, your mission and purpose become clearer. The real takeaway from this book is in the personal call to action each of these individuals developed as part of their recovery and mental health management process. The bravery and resolve it takes to turn one's pain and suffering into action in an effort to support and help others is enormous.

Talking about mental health today isn't just a moment—talking about mental health today is a movement! Now I want to ask YOU to join this movement. Take the time to share mental health resources, to observe and acknowledge mental health specific calendar days, to share your story when you are ready, and call out stigma whenever you see it. Mental health needs more advocates, activists, and champions. I speak for every person featured in this book when I say our collective call to action is to ask you to join us!

I don't think people fully realize how much effort, strength, and courage it takes to pull yourself out of a mentally dark place. So, to anyone suffering who feels invisible and alone, I want you to know:

Your story is far from over, the best parts of your story are yet to come, and that you are NEVER alone.

Acknowledgements

Writing this book and knowing these amazing people featured in it has been one of the most impactful experiences of my life. These shared stories are some of the most authentic and real representations of what is going on in our country concerning mental illness, addiction, and recovery.

It takes great courage and strength to find one's path to wellness. Through story, this incredible group of people share their resiliency, grace, and unconquerable spirit with the world. The contributors in this book are survivors. How do you thank people for sharing their grief, pain, and sadness? Honestly, the answer is you can't. I can only say, from the bottom of my heart, thank you!

I want to thank my wife Marlize and son Noah for their patience, love, and understanding as I manage my mental health every day. I've been speaking about mental health, including my own challenges, nonstop for the past few years. Being vulnerable and sharing one's personal story, thoughts, and fears with crowds over and over again can take its toll on your mental health. My family has been supportive beyond measure and helped me through the emotionally draining times. This book is for them; their unconditional love and encouragement gave me the strength to write it. I love you both.

I want like to express my gratitude to the board of directors and executive leadership at Gracepoint and the Gracepoint Foundation for allowing me to take on this worthwhile project, their encouragement and support to write this book, and the opportunity they gave me to share it with the world. Special thank you to my Foundation colleague Ashley Schlechty for helping me research and edit the early drafts of the book.

Sharing stories may be the most important thing we can do to not only help ourselves, but to also help others. THANK YOU to every mental health care professional, care giver, and advocate who inspired this book—keep sharing your story!

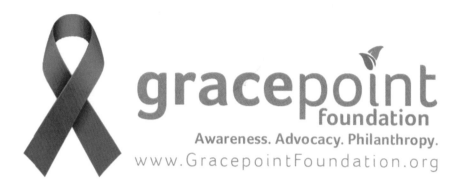

100% of the proceeds from the sale of this book will benefit the Gracepoint Foundation.

About the Gracepoint Foundation

The mission of the Gracepoint Foundation is to raise mental health awareness, financial support, and promote the programs and services of Gracepoint. The Foundation is committed to supporting a strong mental health care system through education, advocacy, and building strong community partnerships.

Gracepoint is the leading behavioral health service provider in Tampa Bay and serves as the behavioral health emergency room for Hillsborough County. Gracepoint impacts the lives of more than 30,000 individuals seeking mental health, addiction treatment, and medical services each year. The mission of Gracepoint is to immediately respond to all people in order to improve their lives by delivering integrated mental health, substance abuse, and medical care to promote health and wellness.

Gracepoint serves the community through a wide range of programs and services. Providing both crisis inpatient and outpatient mental health care for children and adults. Other programs include; behavioral health treatment, substance abuse treatment, supportive and affordable housing, homeless services, family support services, and case management.

Taking care of the wellbeing of our patients and families is at the heart of Gracepoint's work. Gracepoint supports those who are confronting a significant social or mental health challenge in life and your support aids our effort in providing positive mental health and wellness throughout our community.

With the purchase of this book, your support helps provide access to critical services to those having a behavioral health crisis. THANK YOU for making a difference in a life of a child...a family...and a survivor in our community.

An Open Letter to Anyone Struggling Right Now:

You probably feel like you're the only one struggling with this—like everyone else has it all together. They don't. I know you don't want other people to suffer, but maybe that will make you feel less alone.

You've done hard things before—even when you felt like you couldn't, even when you didn't want to, even when it wasn't fair. You did the hard thing and you'll do it again, this time.

You have more resources than you may realize in this moment. There are people who care about you and want you to succeed. There are skills inside of you that may just be covered up by all of the noise. Try to remember those people, places, and things that seem to always help you when things get hard.

Remember, things never stay the same forever. They may not get better right away but they'll get easier and clearer. You will get stronger. You will find your way through.

What you're feeling is real, even if other people can't see it. Validate the feeling and then compare it to the other facts you have. Look for the shades of gray.

When things feel too heavy, take it minute by minute. You don't need to make any decisions right now. When you're ready, you will.

Whitney Goodman, LMFT
Licensed Psychotherapist
Instagram: @sitwithwhit